THE HOLISTIC DOG

A Complete Guide to Natural Health Care

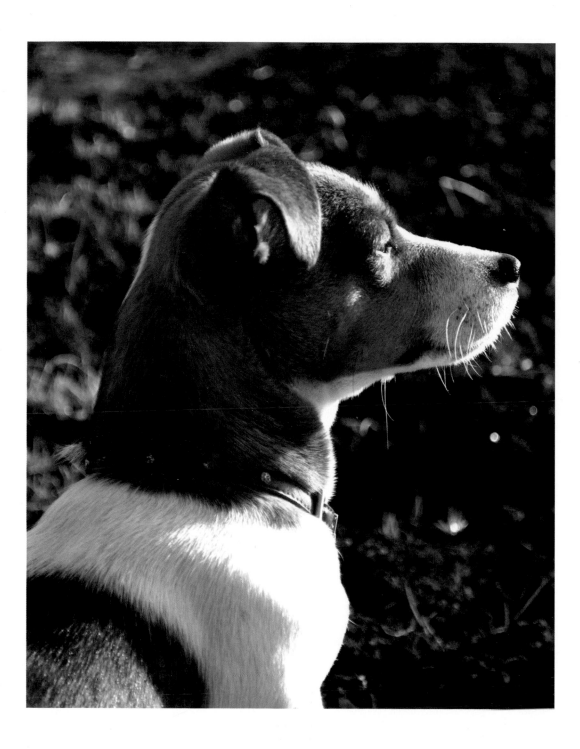

THE HOLISTIC DOG

A Complete Guide to Natural Health Care

Holly Mash

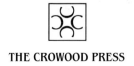

THE CROWOOD PRESS

First published in 2011 by
The Crowood Press Ltd
Ramsbury, Marlborough
Wiltshire SN8 2HR

www.crowood.com

British Library Cataloguing-in-Publication Data
A catalogue record for this book is available from the British
Library.

ISBN 978 1 84797 267 5

Disclaimer
The author and publisher do not accept any responsibility in any
manner whatsoever for any error or omission, or any loss, damage,
injury, adverse outcome, or liability of any kind incurred as a result
of the use of any of the information contained in this book, or
reliance upon it. If in doubt about any aspect of holistic treatment,
readers are advised to seek professional advice.

For simplicity, throughout this book dogs have been referred
to as 'he'.

This book is dedicated to my family.

Typeset by Jean Cussons Typesetting, Diss, Norfolk
Printed and bound in China by Leo Paper Products Ltd.

CONTENTS

PREFACE

I graduated from Veterinary School in 2001 without once being introduced, in any formal way, to complementary medicine. My interest grew from when I worked in a holistic veterinary practice in Sydney and saw first-hand the amazing results of the various treatments on offer at this unique practice. Owners and vets sat on cushions and rugs on the floor of the consulting room with their pets, which were having acupuncture or chiropractic treatment. There were shelves full of strange-smelling herbal medicines from all over the world, and on the walls were charts with intriguing symbols and acupuncture points marked on them. It was while in Australia that I studied Traditional Chinese Medicine and have been practising acupuncture ever since.

Back in the UK, I continued my training in homeopathic medicine at Oxford and Bristol, and am now myself a veterinary tutor on the Bristol course. Studying the various holistic therapies gave me the foundations for a completely new way of interacting with and understanding my patients. I can now appreciate the significance of very subtle symptoms and behaviours that owners tell me about, that I may not have picked up on, or understood the relevance of, before. If an owner tells me that their dog's diarrhoea came on after it was frightened by fireworks, I know that he may very well be helped by the homeopathic remedy Gelsemium (which is for diarrhoea after a shock). Equally, I can now make a link between itchy skin, constipation and irritable behaviour, as all these can be signs of liver qi disturbance in Traditional Chinese Medicine. Every day in my practice I see how my patients benefit from complementary treatments. Dogs with kennel cough don't have to have antibiotics; instead they have marshmallow and Echinacea, while older patients with arthritis are helped by devil's claw or acupuncture, and a daily tonic of Gingko biloba can help with senility. I now have a much greater range tools from which I can choose to treat my patients – and in this book I'm aiming to share the best ones with you.

Over the past few years as 'agony aunt' for *Your Dog* magazine, I have got to know the common problems that dog owners can face. This book is my chance to give them some answers. I wrote this book with the intention of sharing my experience and knowledge, giving owners enough information to have the confidence to be able to offer their dogs a solid foundation in holistic health care. Hopefully you can inspire others as you learn!

Holly Mash, 2011

1 INTRODUCING COMPLEMENTARY THERAPIES

When the minds of the people are closed and wisdom is locked out, they remain tied to disease.

The Yellow Emperor's Classic of Medicine *(220 BC)*

HOLISTIC MEDICINE

'The whole is more than the sum of its parts,' said the Greek philosopher Aristotle, neatly describing the general principle of holism: the idea that all the properties of a given system, in this case medicine, cannot be determined or explained by its component parts alone. Instead, the system as a whole is vital in determining how the parts behave. Therefore in holistic veterinary medicine we consider the whole of each patient, not just the symptom or condition the animal has presented with.

Mind and body

The interrelationship between mind and body has been accepted for centuries in traditional forms of medicine all over the world. In modern veterinary practice it is most easily compared to a branch of medicine called psychoneuroendocrino-immunology (PNEI). This investigates the links between an animal's mind (psycho), its nervous and hormonal systems (neuro-endocrine), and its immune system. In-

depth consultation, usually taking an hour or more, is an important part of most forms of holistic medicine. Your dog's family background, past and present medical history, as well as his diet and daily routine, will all be explored and discussed. The holistic vet will also ask you about your dog's personality and any

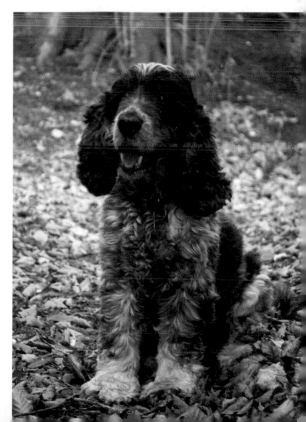

Holistic medicine considers the mind and body as a whole.

individualizing characteristics of his presenting complaint. The details of any diagnostic tests that have been performed may also be of assistance. Finally, as well as observing him carefully throughout the consultation, the vet will also perform a full physical examination of your dog. Holistic medicine understands the strong link between physical and emotional health. It is precisely this consideration of the patient as more than just the sum of its parts that is the key to holistic treatments such as homeopathy and acupuncture. Holistic medicine can therefore be described as treatment of the patient rather than the disease. A holistic approach to healing recognizes that the emotional, mental, spiritual and physical elements of each individual comprise a totality, and it aims to treat the whole patient in this context. It concentrates on the cause of the illness as well as the symptoms.

INTEGRATED HEALTH CARE

What we call conventional veterinary treatment is of course a vital part of our armoury of therapeutic options for your dog. How else apart from surgery are we going to fix his broken leg or neuter him? Indeed, antibiotics are often crucial in helping us combat otherwise life-threatening infections. The aim of 'integrated veterinary medicine' is to use each form of treatment, whether it is herbal, homeopathic, acupuncture, antibiotics or surgery, where it is most appropriate. By widening the scope of possible treatment options for your dog, he will have a greater range of healing possibilities in any given circumstance. With an increasing number of disease-causing organisms becoming resistant to modern drugs, and a growing number of chronic conditions

affecting today's dogs, it is little wonder that there is a shift towards holistic and natural treatment. This is indeed the future for health care for your dog in the twenty-first century. The key to integrated medicine is to use complementary and conventional medicine in conjunction wherever possible. For example, using a homeopathic remedy to speed up healing after orthopaedic surgery has been performed to fix a fractured leg; or using Bach Flower remedies alongside behavioural modification techniques. However, don't forget that all of the complementary therapies outlined here are also complete healing systems in their own right and in many cases will be best suited as the sole form of holistic treatment for your dog.

This chapter will review the most widely available and commonly used complementary treatments, explaining how they work and when they will be most useful. This will help you to know which particular complementary treatment will be best suited to your dog in a given situation.

HOMEOPATHY

Homeopathy is a system of medicine that stimulates the body's own self-healing mechanisms. It is based on the principle that 'like cures like', which has been called the 'law of similars'. This theory dates back to the days of Hippocrates and the Ancient Greeks in the fifth century BCE ('the majority of maladies can be cured by the same things that caused them'). However, it was only when the German physician Dr Samuel Hahnemann formulated it as a complete system of medicine in its own right in the early nineteenth century that homeopathy as we know it today was born.

How does it work?

Homeopathy acknowledges that the body has a natural self-healing mechanism, called the 'vital force'. This can be considered as the energy in every living thing that regulates the body and maintains health. Homeopathic remedies act to stimulate the vital force and restore health in a gentle and natural manner. The following are the most important principles in homeopathic medicine.

The law of similars

Diseases are treated with remedies that in a healthy individual would produce symptoms similar to those that they are used to treat. For example, Allium Cepa, the homeopathic remedy made from red onion, is commonly used to treat symptoms of streaming eyes and nose – the same signs that you get when you slice a red onion. One way of understanding how homeopathic remedies stimulate self-healing is to compare them to how a tuning fork works. When the correct remedy is given to a patient it will resonate with his body and help it to re-tune back to its normal, healthy frequency. The principle of 'like cures like' is at the heart of homeopathic treatment because only the most similarly matched homeopathic remedy will resonate with the body and stimulate healing in this way. This is the reason behind the lengthy and detailed taking of a case history. To make the best 'match' between symptoms and remedy, in other words the most effective prescription, the homeopath needs to know all about your dog and his unique set of symptoms. Then, armed with this information, they will consult their materia medica, books that describe the healing powers of each remedy, and through this process of analysis, called 'repertor-ization', they will be able to find the remedy that most exactly matches your dog's symptoms.

The minimum effective dose

Homeopathic remedies are mainly derived from plants, for example Arnica and Calendula, but others come from minerals, and others still from animal sources. A process called 'potentization' manufactures them. This consists of serially diluting the active component in a solution, and vigorously agitating it at each stage. This process of potentization results in a remedy that is at once energetically active, 'potent', but also highly diluted. The 'potency' is a measure of the 'strength' of a homeopathic remedy. It is denoted by a 'c' or 'x' after a number, for example 30c or 6x. These letters relate to the two most common potency scales used in homeopathy, that of the centesimal scale (c), where there has been a dilution of one in a hundred at each stage in the manufacture, and the decimal scale (x), where the dilution is one in ten. However paradoxical it sounds, the more dilute the remedy, the more potent it becomes. For example, a 30c remedy is stronger than a 12c remedy. This is because, although it is more diluted, the remedy has also gone through more of the activating 'sucussions' in its manufacture. The remedies range from low potency 6c to high potency 200c and 1M (a different scale altogether, used for high-potency remedies). For most everyday use of homeopathy for your dog, you would be using 12c or 30c potency remedies.

Treating the individual, not the disease

The homeopath will always need to build up a complete picture of each individual patient through taking a detailed case history, and by careful observation during the consultation. They will ask about the history of the illness or condition and when it started, as well as about your dog's medical history apart from his current complaint. They will ask about his family background, and where you got him. You will also be asked details about his everyday routines, his character and personality, and any factors that make your dog's presenting complaint either better or worse. No detail is too insignificant for the veterinary homeopath, as the most unusual symptom or characteristic of your dog may be the key that helps them to find the most suitable remedy for him.

Obstacles to cure
This is another guiding principle in homeopathy and means that any factor in the patient's life that may be hampering the action of the homeopathic remedies

should be removed whenever possible. This relates to the holistic idea that unless contributory factors that affect your dog's overall health, such as nutrition, vaccination, environmental and emotional factors, are addressed, the homeopathic treatment cannot work to its full potential.

What is it used for?
Homeopathy is a system of medicine in its own right, suitable for treating a wide range of conditions, from the sudden to the long-standing. Home treatment is valuable for a range of mild ailments and as a first aid measure. For example, using arnica for bruises, calendula cream for cuts and grazes, and ruta for strains and sprains (*see* Chapter 9). However, in-depth consultation and referral to a veterinary homeopath will be suitable for ongoing or chronic conditions such as allergies, epilepsy or cancer. Finally,

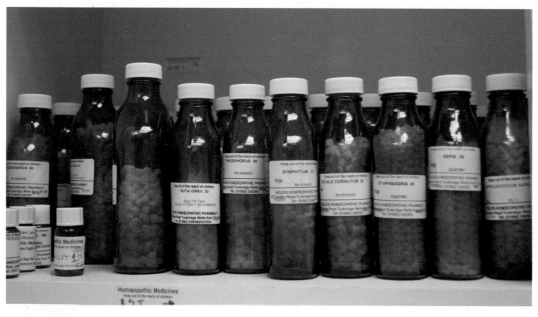

Homeopathic remedies.

homeopathy should be considered as a treatment option in conditions where conventional medicine may not be possible, or indeed where there is no other treatment available.

How to administer and store remedies

Homeopathic medicines are called 'remedies' and each remedy can be bought in whichever formulation is easiest for you to give to your dog: tablets, liquids or powders. They are best given to your dog between meals, in other words not with his food, nor within about twenty minutes of any other medicines. Careful storage of remedies is important. Keep them away from any highly aromatic substances (such as mint, lavender or garlic), magnetic fields, electromagnetic radiation (such as mobile phones and computers), as well as extreme temperatures and direct sunlight. You are also recommended not to handle homeopathic remedies; try and tip tablets directly from the lid of the container into your dog's mouth. These special recommendations are given because the subtle healing properties of the remedies can be easily overpowered and negated. However, if you are having real problems getting your dog to take a homeopathic remedy, then it can be given with a little plain food.

Dosage

Most commonly indicated remedies that you may have reason to use for your dog will be 12c or 30c potency. One pill or tablet is one dose, and in liquid formulations one dose is one to two drops. It is how often you give the remedy and the potency that you use, rather than the number of tablets or drops given at any one time, that is the key to homeopathic dosing. Homeopathic remedies are always given one dose at a time, waiting for the response in the patient after each one. A general rule of thumb is to match how often you give the remedy to how quickly the problem started, dosing more frequently for sudden onset complaints and less often for long-standing ones. The other important thing to understand is to stop dosing when you see a change in the patient's symptoms – whether this is a mental and emotional improvement or a physical one. This is an indication that your dog's self-healing mechanisms have been stimulated into action and the remedy has done its job. You may well see an improvement in your dog's mental and emotional state before you see an improvement in his physical symptoms.

Integrated treatment

Side effects to homeopathic treatment are rare. However, you should be aware of the possibility of what is called an aggravation. This is when your dog's symptoms get temporarily worse immediately following the first one or two doses of a homeopathic remedy. It is not common and usually means that he was given too high a potency or that he is especially sensitive to the remedy. If your dog suffers from an aggravation do not give him any further doses. The symptoms will usually settle within twenty-four to forty-eight hours, and then he will start to get better.

If your dog is taking any conventional medications at the same time that he is having homeopathic treatment, it will be important to follow the advice of your veterinary homeopath. He should be receiving integrated care, which means that your dog is given the best and most appropriate form of treatment for any given condition.

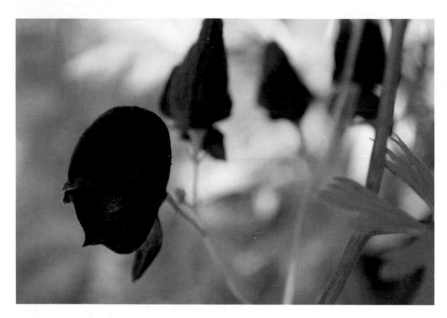

Aconitum Napellus (Monkshood), the homeopathic remedy for shock.

How to find a qualified practitioner
Fully qualified homeopathic vets will have the letters VetMFHom after their name. The governing body for veterinary homeopaths is the Faculty of Homeopathy (*see* Useful Addresses, page 173).

HERBAL MEDICINE

Herbalism is the most widely used and ancient form of medical practice still in use today. It has been integral to the medical traditions of cultures in China and India as well as Western Europe for thousands of years. One of the earliest records of animals being treated with herbs was in the Ayurvedic *Nakul Samhita*, a treatise concerning horses and elephants written between 4500 and 1600 BCE. Since then, veterinary botanical medicine has grown and spread, and as recently as the 1960s herbal formulas were listed in veterinary textbooks and considered as orthodox medicine. Currently there is a worldwide

drive to source plants with medicinal properties. Unfortunately, we are frequently too late, as they are lost forever due to environmental destruction and the loss of the indigenous peoples that have the knowledge of their healing powers.

How does it work?
With the majority of our modern drugs, including veterinary ones, derived from plants, Nature's healing properties are well known. Herbs provide us with a great variety of pharmacologically active ingredients, called phytochemicals, ranging from laxatives and purgatives to astringents and sedatives. They are also categorized in Western herbal medicine according to their action on the body, some acting on a particular organ, others as whole-body tonics. In addition, herbs can act to help the body to detoxify itself through the promotion of urination (diuretics), bowel movements (purgatives), or to support the immune system

(adaptogens). Other cultures will have different ways of categorizing herbal medicines, but the uses will be the same.

Nature's medicine chest provides the basis for most medicines we use today. For example, the active principle in the painkiller morphine comes from the poppy, that of the heart drug digitalis from the foxglove, and, more recently, an important cancer drug has been derived from the periwinkle. However, these pharmaceutical medicines will only contain a single active component, or extract, of the plant, whereas in herbal medicine the whole thing is used. This is because the other parts of the plant provide important nutrients and phyto-chemicals that support the rest of the body. Thus, using the whole leaf, root, flower or seed ensures that the variety of compounds that occur naturally in the plant are available for the body to use, giving it a holistic action. One such example is the dandelion. Dandelion leaf is rich in minerals, including potassium, so that when it is used as a diuretic it naturally replenishes the body with this mineral, whereas the diuretic drug, with its narrow scope of action, would not.

What is it used for?
Herbs can be used effectively as medicines in their own right, or in conjunction with conventional drugs. When they are used in a holistic manner herbs act to gently stimulate the body's self-healing mechanisms. Alternatively, herbs can be used in a superficial manner, to get rid of symptoms without addressing the underlying cause. Finally, it shouldn't be

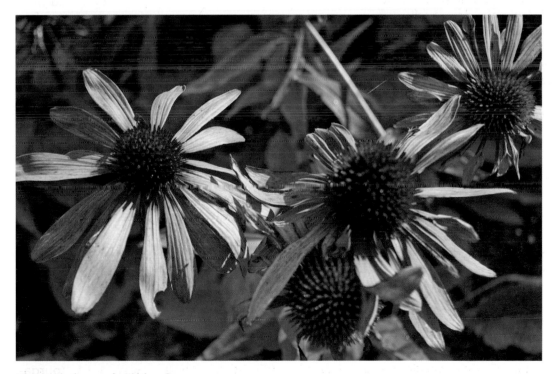

The herbal remedy Echinacea.

forgotten that herbs are also foods; their culinary qualities are just as important as their medicinal ones. A wide range of herbs can be used as dietary supplements to provide your dog with minerals, vitamins, fatty acids and other important nutritional components. Commonly used nutritive herbs include spirulina, nettle, dandelion leaf and alfalfa.

Administration of herbal medicines
Herbs can be given to your dog in a variety of different ways. You might pick them fresh from the garden to sprinkle on his food, or use dried formulations, tinctures, tablets, capsules, ointments or infusions. Be aware that a herb's physical and chemical composition determines how it needs to be prepared and administered as a medicine. As every herb is different, this will of course affect how you can use it. For instance, it would be ineffective to make an infusion of a herb whose main active constituent was not water-soluble. Another important factor is that you should source any herbal product from a reputable and established company that has rigorous quality-control measures. This will ensure that any problems associated with contamination and wrongly identified herbs are avoided. You should also check that your herbs are derived from sustainable sources, rather than wild plants, and are organically grown and naturally harvested. Always consult a specialist herbal vet before starting your dog on any herbal supplement or medicine. That way you won't get the wrong herb or the wrong dose, and you will know that it won't interfere with any other medicines he may be taking. This is very important.

Fresh herbs
Many fresh culinary herbs, such as parsley, thyme and garlic, can be added directly to your dog's food using just a little, such as a chopped teaspoonful, at once. You can also make an infusion from freshly picked herbs. These can often be the best medicines; when the plant is freshly picked it still full of its active, health-giving ingredients.

Tablets and capsules
These will contain either powdered dried herbs, or extracts, so dosage will vary depending on the amount of active ingredient they contain. Products formulated especially for dogs will have the dosage on the label; otherwise your veterinary herbalist will guide you. Do not assume that human products can simply be given to your dog at a reduced dosage; this is not always the case. As well as possibly giving him the wrong dose, your dog may also be unable to digest a tablet or capsule that was manufactured for human consumption. Therefore, using a human preparation for your dog may be ineffective as well as potentially harmful.

Infusion
Infusions are like herbal teas. They are made by adding one teaspoon of the dried herb, or one tablespoon of fresh, to a cup of water that is just off the boil, allowing it to steep for fifteen minutes, and then straining it. However, infusions can also be left to steep overnight for added potency. They should be made freshly each day and can be added, once cooled, to your dog's food. Give him a little (one tablespoonful) at each meal or offer it as a broth. Infusions can also be useful skin and coat rinses. Remember, however, that they are only effective if the herb's active constituents are water-soluble, so you will need to do your

homework on the given herb. When using dried herbs, store them in an airtight container and remember that they will lose their potency over time (renewing annually is recommended).

Decoction

This is like an infusion but is used for the hard parts of the plant, such as roots or bark. It is made by simmering herbs in water for fifteen or twenty minutes, then leaving them to soak for several hours (or overnight). Like the infusion, they can be added to your dog's food.

Tinctures

These potent herbal medicines are made by extracting and concentrating the active constituents from the herb using alcohol. They are very concentrated forms of the herb, so doses will only usually be a few drops. Due to the alcohol content tinctures may be unpalatable for dogs. However, when they are diluted with water and added to their food, most dogs will take them without a problem. You can get glycerin-based tinctures, with no alcohol; these can be helpful if your dog won't take the standard tincture.

Creams

Calendula, comfrey, echinacea and other herbs can be made into creams and ointments by macerating the fresh plant and combining the juice with a base cream such as vitamin E. There are many commercially available herbal creams, but do check the ingredients carefully before you use them on your dog. This is because he is likely to lick some of it off, and you need to make sure it is safe if he does.

Dosage

Because herbs can be potentially danger-
ous, it is vital to use the correct dosage. Always begin with small doses, and see how your dog tolerates them, before increasing to the required dose of any herbal medicine. It is common for several herbs to be used together as a preparation, as they work synergistically, enhancing one another's action and also minimizing the potential for side effects. Unless you are using a product made specifically for dogs, with guidelines on the label, you will always need to seek the advice of a veterinary herbalist before using any herbal preparation for your dog. Different preparations of the same herb can contain different amounts of active constituent, depending on when and where it was harvested, the type of plant, and the part used; each of these variables can alter its strength and potency. Herbs are generally not intended for long-term use, as some that are beneficial when given for a few days or weeks can be toxic if given over the long term.

Self-medicating

Animals instinctively know how to medicate themselves from wild plants. There is a whole area of science devoted to the study of how animals self-medicate, called zoopharmacognosy. Wild animals have been shown to know instinctively not only which plants will help them, but how much of the plant to eat, as some are poisonous at higher doses. Dogs chew grass (couch grass, or 'dog grass') when they are feeling nauseous and want to vomit. Indeed, the story goes that the Greek god of medicine, Asclepius, said that he admired dogs the most out of all animals because they knew and used herbs to prevent and cure all the ailments of the canine race. So plant some herbs in your garden and

HERBALISM AND HOMEOPATHY

These two forms of holistic medicine are often confused. This usually stems from the fact that many homeopathic remedies are derived from plants that are also used in herbal medicine. However, they are very different healing systems. Homeopathy is an energy-based system, while herbal medicine uses measurable amounts of the herb in its medicines. If you go wrong with homeopathy, usually the worst that can happen is that your dog does not improve. But if you use the wrong herbs or the wrong dose, then there is the potential for toxicity. That's why it is essential to realize that these are two different branches of holistic medicine.

allow your dog to choose them himself as and when he feels that he needs them. A few herbs to start with are couch grass, chickweed, dandelion and burdock. You will be surprised to notice that he will pick out different grasses to chew on in order to medicate himself; most domestic dogs have not lost this instinct.

Integrated treatment

Seeking the advice of a specialist vet is always essential when using any herbal medicine for your dog. This is because any herb has the potential to be harmful as well as healing. Herbs can cause side effects, such as vomiting or diarrhoea, or your dog may have an allergic reaction to them. Herbs can also interact with certain conventional medications and other supplements your dog may be taking. All of these are reasons for veterinary guidance.

How to find a qualified practitioner

The British Association of Veterinary Herbalists represents veterinary surgeons trained in herbal medicine (*see* Useful Addresses, page 173).

ACUPUNCTURE

Acupuncture originated several thousand years ago in East Asia, as a form of Traditional Chinese Medicine (TCM). Ancient records and clay models of horses with acupuncture points marked on them have been traced to this period. Western civilizations gradually adopted acupuncture practice until it gained major popularity as a complementary veterinary practice in the 1970s, with the establishment of the International Veterinary Acupuncture Society (IVAS).

How does it work?

Acupuncture is defined as the insertion of fine needles into specific points on the body. How acupuncture works can be explained by two very different theories, the Western and the Traditional Chinese. According to the Western understanding of acupuncture, the insertion of needles triggers the release of a complex cascade of chemicals in the body, and causes a modification of the pain pathways in the brain and spinal cord. Both of these effects result in pain relief for the patient. In addition there are more generalized effects of acupuncture needling on the body. It has a regulatory effect on the dog's nervous and hormonal systems, as well as his circulatory, digestive and immune functions. Over the past thirty years there has been much research into acupuncture, leading to several well-accepted neurophysiological models for its mode of action. Finally, on a microscopic level it has been shown that acupuncture points can be differentiated from the surrounding skin. They have an increased number of nerve endings, blood vessels and immune system tissue, as well as a lowered electrical resistance.

In Traditional Chinese Medicine, acupuncture is just one element in a range of therapies used to restore health, including herbal medicine, breathing and movement exercises (Qi gung and Tai Qi), and attention to diet. Fundamental to the TCM understanding of health and disease is the concept of a vital energy called qi (pronounced chee), which flows through the body along channels called meridians. Qi is maintained by yin and yang, the equal and opposite forces whose perfect balance keeps the body in harmony and health. Pain and disease are seen as a blockage of qi. Acupuncture points are the places along the meridians where the body's qi energy can be tapped into by the insertion of needles. This alters and rebalances the flow of qi, and hence restores health. Traditional Chinese Medicine is based on the Taoist principles of seeing the body as a reflection of the universe. Philosophers understood the interrelationship between the universe and the human body as a continuous cycle of qi. They placed great importance on living a life in harmony with one's environment, balancing the active and the passive, the yin and yang. In the third and fourth centuries BC doctors had to rely on their sense of sight, smell, taste, hearing and touch to diagnose and treat illness. Hence they formulated associations between the seasons, the weather, and the physical lie of the land around them (the hills, mountains and rivers) with the inner workings of the body. This is the basis for the five element theory, a common method of diagnosis and treatment in TCM.

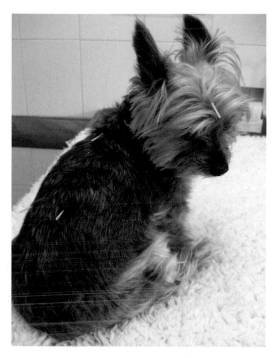

Acupuncture treatment for back pain.

Each acupuncture treatment is tailored to the individual patient, incorporating the use of different points in order to harmonize their specific qi imbalance. Chinese herbs will often be used as part of your dog's TCM treatment alongside his acupuncture.

What is it used for?
Acupuncture is used to provide a natural form of pain relief for many conditions, most commonly those of the musculoskeletal system such as lameness and arthritis. It is also especially helpful for dogs that cannot be given conventional painkillers, or who suffer from their side effects. However, Traditional Chinese Medicine and acupuncture are also a complete medical system in their own right and can therefore be indicated for

the treatment of a wide range of medical problems. These commonly include skin conditions and immune system diseases.

Integrated treatment

Acupuncture is becoming increasingly accepted and integrated into conventional veterinary practice. This is due in large part to the fact that it can be understood within the framework of Western medicine. In other words, you don't have to believe in the concept of qi to be able to explain how it works. Your regular vet may give your dog acupuncture as part of a routine appointment or may refer him to a specialist vet. Acupuncture should not usually be done if your dog is pregnant.

The acupuncture treatment itself consists of the insertion of around eight to twelve ultra-fine, sterile, single-use needles into the skin on various places on your dog's body. He will usually be sitting or lying down for his treatment, and the needles are left in place for between ten and fifteen minutes. In addition to relieving pain, acupuncture also has a sedative action on the body. Some dogs become quite sleepy and tranquil during the session as the needles stimulate the release of natural sedatives into their circulation. Your dog may be a little sleepy or tired for up to twenty-four hours after a treatment, but this is not usually the case.

While some dogs are highly responsive to acupuncture and will show a marked improvement after just a single treatment, the majority of patients need several sessions before a change is seen. Acupuncture is usually done weekly for the first four sessions, reducing in frequency after that, depending on the nature of the condition and the response of the patient. Many elderly, arthritic dogs are treated every four to six weeks

to help them remain comfortable. A minority of dogs can be unresponsive to acupuncture and will not respond to treatment. It is also the case that very anxious dogs and those that do not tolerate handling and examination will not be the best candidates for acupuncture and hence would benefit from a different form of treatment.

How to find a qualified practitioner

Vets trained in acupuncture will usually have gained their qualifications through either the International Veterinary Acupuncture Society (IVAS), in which case they will have a more Traditional Chinese Medicine approach to treatment, or they will have done a course though the Association of British Veterinary Acupuncturists (ABVA) – *see* Useful Addresses, page 173.

VARIATIONS ON ACUPUNCTURE

There are variations on the everyday 'dry needling' technique used in acupuncture that may be more useful in certain situations. Laser acupuncture employs infrared lasers to stimulate acupuncture points, and is a useful technique in dogs that are needle-shy. Electroacupuncture uses a pulse of electric current to stimulate the needles, and is generally used in hospitalized patients. Moxibustion is where a Chinese herb (*Artemisia vulgaris*) is burnt over the acupuncture point; it is most commonly used for elderly patients with sluggish qi. Finally, a technique called aquapuncture, whereby a sterile liquid is injected into acupuncture points, can be used for prolonged stimulation, to treat long-standing pain, for example.

THE BACH FLOWER REMEDIES

The Bach Flower Remedies are a series of thirty-eight flower essences that are used to treat a wide range of emotional or behavioural problems. The best known is Rescue Remedy, used for shock.

How do they work?

The Bach Flower Remedies were developed in the 1930s by Dr Edward Bach (pronounced Batch), a pioneering Harley Street surgeon and homeopath, who wanted to find a gentle and natural way of healing. He sought a simple, safe way to restore harmony in the body through emotional well-being. After many years working with the flowers and trees in the Oxfordshire countryside where he lived, Dr Bach developed his series of flower remedies. They work on the same energetic or vibrational principles as homeopathic remedies and have an effect on the emotional and spiritual levels of the body, to stimulate self-healing. Bach Flower Remedies balance negative emotions, such as grief, anger and frustration, into positive ones, such as happiness and contentment. Each of the thirty-eight remedies helps to deal with a particular negative state of mind. Dr Bach understood the link between stress, emotions and illness when he said that there was no true healing unless there was a change in outlook, peace of mind, and inner happiness. These flower essences do not use the physical material of the plant, like herbal medicines, but rather the essential energy that is found within the flower. It is this that represents their healing quality. Dr Bach's dream was that his system of thirty-eight flower remedies should be easy enough to prescribe and use so that people could use them for everyday situations at home. He wanted to give people the power to heal themselves, their family and friends and those around them. Even though they were developed for use in people, Bach Flower Remedies have been used to treat animals for over fifty years.

Since Dr Bach's day, several different systems of flower essences have been developed and are now used all over the world, from California to Australia. However, it seems most appropriate to use the Bach flower essences on British dogs, as their bodies will be more attuned to the essence of our native wild flowers.

How are they made?

Dr Bach chose only those flowers that grew wild and uncultivated and were non-poisonous; he felt that the strength and purity of the plants was important. This healing energy is extracted by simple methods that are still followed when the essences are made at the Bach Flower Centre today. A glass bowl is filled with pure water, and then the flowers are picked and floated on the water to cover the surface. This must be done on a clear, sunny day when the flowers are in perfect bloom. The bowl is then left in the sunlight for three to four hours and the healing energy within the flowers is transferred into the water. This is then used as the basis of the flower essence, which is preserved in alcohol and bottled into the range that you can buy in most large pharmacies or health food shops. There are now Bach flower essences that are preserved in non-alcoholic media such as glycerin. Similarly there is an alcohol-free Rescue Remedy.

Put yourself in your dog's shoes

When you are using these flower essences for your dog, you have to try

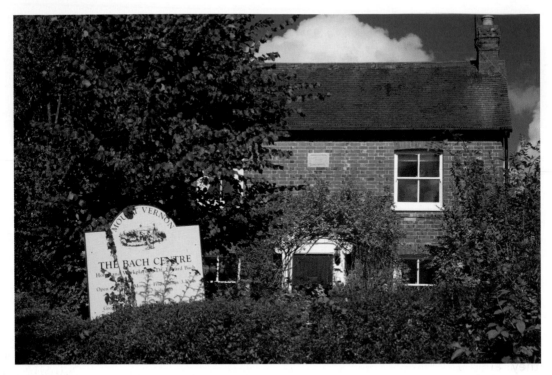

The Bach Centre, home of Dr Edward Bach.

and work out exactly which emotion or emotions he is feeling. This can obviously be a difficult business, as it is all too easy to anthropomorphize and misinterpret his signals. Therefore when we are using these thirty-eight flower remedies for dogs, we need to remember to try and look at the situation from his point of view, and not just prescribe for the natural human emotion in a given situation. For example, think how terrified and panic-stricken dogs can be about having their nails clipped – here a remedy for extreme fear and terror may be applicable. It's also important to realize that there are some negative emotions that Dr Bach identified, such as bitterness and hatred, which we would very rarely attribute to a dog. Therefore animal

treatment with flower essences can be complex and will involve a good insight into your dog's behaviour. If you can't work out what your dog is feeling, or if your combination of flower remedies has not worked in a given situation, you should consult a qualified Bach Flower Animal Practitioner.

What are they used for?
The Bach Flower Remedies are used to treat emotional disturbances in dogs. These can be trauma-related, or anxiety-and-fear based problems. The remedies are often especially helpful for ex-rescue dogs that may have a traumatic past history (*see* Chapter 2). Examples of where Bach Flower Remedies are indicated include helping dogs to adjust to

new situations, such as the arrival of a new baby into the family, or a new pet. They are also used to help ease the transition between life stages, such as weaning, sexual maturity, and ageing. These flower remedies are a useful aid in housetraining a puppy, as well as for calming fears and phobias, such as fear of thunderstorms or fireworks. Bach Flower Remedies can also be used in treating grief states and for anxiety around travel or showing. Rescue Remedy is the best known of the Bach Flower Remedies and is a composite of five flower essences. It can be used to treat the shock and panic that normally arise in any emergency situation.

How to administer
Bach Flower Remedies

Bach flower essences are liquid remedies; they are used diluted and given by mouth, usually on food. If you have seen a Bach Flower practitioner they will have made up a bottle of essences ready for you to use. However, if you are consulting books and prescribing the essences for your dog yourself, you will need to buy the stock bottles of each different flower essence. You then add two drops from the stock bottle of each of your chosen

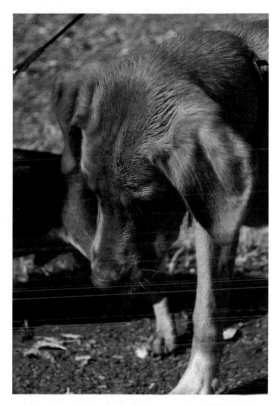

Bach Flower Remedies are used to balance the emotions.

essences (up to a maximum of six different ones), to a thirty or fifty millilitre bottle of spring water. This bottle of diluted essences is what you will use to dose your dog. As it is mainly spring water and does not contain any preservative, your bottle of essences will only remain viable for up to three weeks. At this stage you will either change the combination of flower essences you use, or make him up a new bottle. If you are using a single flower essence, you can administer directly from the stock bottle. When preparing and giving the remedies it is important not to touch the tip of the dropper, to avoid contamination.

POPULAR USES OF BACH FLOWER REMEDIES

Star of Bethlehem: used for the after-effects of shock, useful for rescue dogs.
Mimulus: used to treat fear of fireworks or thunderstorms.
Walnut: used to help your dog adapt to change, such as the arrival of a new baby.

HOW TO USE RESCUE REMEDY

Rescue Remedy can be used to treat shock in a wide range of different situations, from major road traffic accidents to that of nail clipping. You can also use it in anticipation of a traumatic event, dosing your dog before a trip to the vet's for example. In these situations, start giving it to your dog about forty-five minutes before the anticipated event, giving four drops every fifteen minutes. For use after shocks, give four drops every ten to fifteen minutes until your dog appears calmer.

Dosage
The dose of Bach Flower Remedies is four drops at least four times daily. The best way of administering them to your dog is to put them on a little food, such as a treat. Otherwise you can add the four drops to his water bowl and he will get the doses as he drinks throughout the day. It is preferable to offer your dog his doses via a treat, in other words separately from his meal, so that he has a choice in taking the flower remedy. Dosing will be daily for as long as required; however, you should review after about three weeks to see how they have helped. Drops should never be administered directly from the glass dropper into your dog's mouth, as this is potentially dangerous. When dosing by mouth is difficult, or if you do not want to give your dog anything to eat, rubbing the drops onto the skin at the base of the ears is another option. They will be absorbed more slowly than if given by mouth, but this is an effective alternative when regular dosing is not possible.

Integrated treatment
Bach flower essences are highly user-friendly and are a great tool for you to use at home. They are safe, do not have any side effects, and can usually be used alongside conventional medicines without interference.

How to find a qualified practitioner
A Bach Foundation Registered Animal Practitioner (BFRAP) will be fully qualified to treat emotional and behavioural problems in animals using the Bach Flower Remedies (*see* Useful Addresses, page 173).

TELLINGTON TOUCH

The Tellington TTouch or TTouch is a way of healing and training your dog using gentle and directed finger touches anywhere on his body. Your dog can benefit from TTouch to help with a great range of behavioural problems and to assist in training. Because it is so simple and intuitive, TTouch is a popular method of hands-on treatment for dogs.

How does it work?
Tellington Touch is a way of working non-habitually with an animal's body to create new behaviour patterns. It works on the understanding that the body's tissues store memories of pain, disease and fear and that the TTouches help to release these, facilitating healing and relaxation. Emotional and mental well-being and balance are intimately linked to physical balance. By removing tension in your dog's body using TTouch, his new, relaxed posture will help him to behave in a calmer and more controlled manner. TTouch was first developed in the 1970s by the Canadian horse trainer Linda Tellington-Jones, who based it on the

human bodywork therapy called Feldenkrais. It involves using repeated, random massage movements on the body to stimulate your dog's nervous system and restore the connections and awareness between mind and body. The understanding is that the brain pays better attention to these unfamiliar sensations and thus TTouch allows change to take place on all levels, from the mental to the physical. The related `ground-work` techniques are an integral part of the TTouch method, and involve the use of special balance leads and harnesses. Working your dog over poles and through zig-zags helps him to focus and ground himself, again achieving the connection between mind and body.

Hands-on healing

Hands-on healing has a history going back thousands of years and has been practised by different cultures all over the world. Holding our hands over a place on the body that hurts is one of our most basic instincts. Thus TTouch is tapping into this primal instinct to heal. When you use TTouch on your dog you are establishing a non-verbal communication that strengthens the bond between you, and increases trust.

What is it used for?

TTouch can be a very effective way of treating a wide range of behavioural and emotional problems. For example, it can be used to calm dogs in stressful situations, relieve discomfort and aid healing after surgery or injury, and help a fearful dog become more confident. TTouch can help to address problems such as noise phobia, separation anxiety, and fear (which can be anything from fear of the vet to fear of thunder or fireworks). TTouch can also help dogs that do not

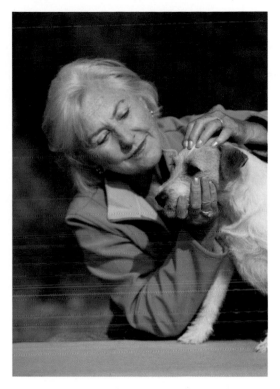

Linda Tellington-Jones gives TTouch to a dog. (Photo: Gabriele Metz/Kosmos, from Tellington-Training für Hunde, *Kosmos Verlag)*

travel well and those that hate being groomed or having their nails clipped. It is also an invaluable aid to training or obedience problems. In addition it can be used to help stimulate wound healing and in rehabilitation after injury or an operation. TTouch helps to increase circulation, reduce stiffness, promote a feeling of calm and relaxation, change a habitual behaviour, increase self-confidence, and release tension.

Your first move: 'The Clouded Leopard'

To do 'TTouch', cup your hand softly with the thumb and fingers resting lightly on your dog. Use your middle three fingers to make a circular movement as if you are pushing the skin around an imaginary clock-face. Start at the six o'clock position and move the skin in a complete circle and a quarter, clockwise. You can make the circle as large or as small as you want, but the movement should be smooth and flowing. Press just firmly enough to gently slide the skin over the tissues beneath, hold it for a moment and then gently move your hand and repeat this circular TTouch on another area. Avoid making repeated circles on the same spot. This simple TTouch movement is called 'The Clouded Leopard', signifying softness and strength, and you can use it all over your dog's body. Continue for as long as he is enjoying it, paying attention at all times to how he is responding to it. Stop if he moves away, and if he fidgets when you work on a particular part of his body go back to a place where the contact was more acceptable. Your dog may only sit quietly for a few moments to start with, until he gets used to the feeing of TTouch. A variation on the above technique, called the Llama TTouch, where you use the back of your hand, is especially good for anxious dogs and those that do not like being touched.

Integrated treatment

One of the major benefits of this form of treatment is that TTouch can be readily learnt and used on your dog every day at home, and you don't need any specialist equipment. It can be used as a complement to any other treatment that your dog is having, or it can be used on its own. It causes no harm, and there are no side effects.

How to find a qualified practitioner

Although the basic techniques can quite easily be learnt, for serious problems you will need the expertise of a trained TTouch practitioner (*see* Useful Addresses, page 173).

CHIROPRACTIC

Chiropractic treatment adjusts misaligned joints throughout the body, paying particular attention to the spine and pelvis. It is based on the philosophy that the spinal column is integral to the health of the whole body due to its relationship with the nervous system. Therefore if the vertebrae are even subtly misaligned, they will be putting pressure on the nerves of the spinal cord, and hence having a detrimental effect on the functioning of the entire body. The McTimoney method is a particularly gentle method of chiropractic treatment that is used on animals.

How does it work?

The word chiropractic comes from the Greek word *chiropraktikos*, meaning effective treatment by hand. The McTimoney method was developed by the British chiropractor John McTimoney in the 1950s.

It is well suited for use on animals because its gentle nature makes it ethical and respectful. During the treatment the chiropractor will carefully assess the exact orientation of each vertebrae along your dog's spine, and will correct any deviation with very gentle, subtle and extremely quick movements using their fingers. Thus they will work their way from your dog's head to his tail, correcting and adjusting as they go. Most dogs will need a slight adjustment, even if they seem perfectly sound and healthy. By adjusting the misaligned joints throughout the whole body, with special

The McTimoney chiropractic method is particularly gentle for dogs.

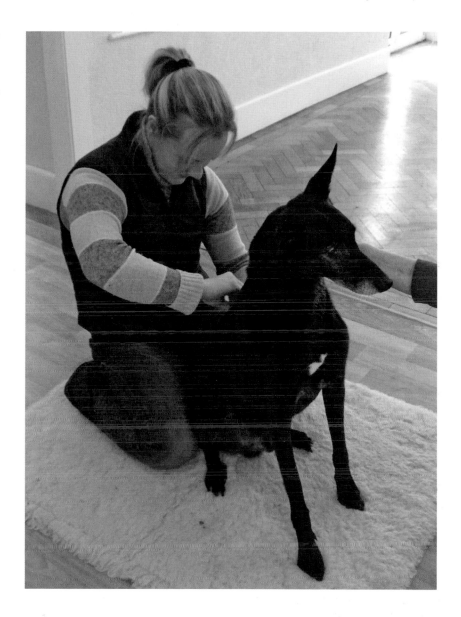

attention to the spine and pelvis, chiropractic treatment can restore health, soundness and normal functioning in a holistic manner. If your dog has been lame or stiff for a while, he may need a few treatments in order for his body to be able to retain the new pattern of alignment.

What is it used for?

Your dog can benefit from chiropractic adjustment if he has any back, neck or other musculoskeletal pain or stiffness. This can come about through twisting, or jumping into or out of the car, or from a falls or another trauma. Or he may just be old and arthritic. Some breeds of dog, especially those with longer backs, or performance and agility dogs, will be more prone to these problems. Indeed agility and working dogs can benefit from regular sessions with the chiropractor to help prevent potential problems before they arise. It may also be used to maximize performance in dogs by allowing the body to work at its optimal level biomechanically. In addition, because spinal nerves affect all the organs, glands and tissues of the body, chiropractic adjustment has a wider scope of action than simply those affecting your dog's mobility. The aim of chiropractic treatment is to relieve pain and discomfort and increase mobility and flexibility in the body, as well as being a boost to overall health.

Integrated treatment

Your dog may have chiropractic treatment as the sole form of therapy or it may be used in combination with, for example, acupuncture, or as part of a rehabilitation programme alongside physiotherapy. According to chiropractic philosophy, the treatment should be used to maintain health, and not just to treat symptoms. This is why it is considered part of a health maintenance regime for many dogs.

How to find a qualified practitioner

Animal chiropractors can only work by referral from your vet. The McTimoney Chiropractic Association (MCA) was the first, and remains one of the only, chiropractic associations to train and qualify chiropractors to treat animals (*see* Useful Addresses, page 173). All animal chiropractors are initially qualified in human chiropractic and do a postgraduate qualification in animal manipulation.

THE LAW AND COMPLEMENTARY THERAPY PRACTITIONERS

According to the Royal College of Veterinary Surgeons' guide to professional conduct, treatment by acupuncture, aromatherapy, homeopathy or any other complementary therapy may only be given by a veterinary surgeon who has undergone training in these procedures. At present, it is illegal for them to be given by practitioners who are not veterinary surgeons. The only exceptions to this, that allow non-veterinary surgeons to treat animals, are physiotherapists, osteopaths and chiropractors. However, these physical manipulation therapists will still be working under the guidance of a veterinary surgeon, who will refer the animal to them for treatment. You can legally treat your own dog provided you do not cause him 'unnecessary suffering'.

What is a referral?

A referral is the process by which your vet sends your dog to a specialist vet, such as one trained in a complementary therapy. A referral will usually be necessary for any of the specialist therapies outlined in this chapter, with the exception of Bach Flower Remedies and TTouch which, in some cases, you may practise on your own dog at home. The process of referral generally involves your vet completing a referral form and sending this, together with your dog's full medical history, to the specialist vet. They in turn send a report back to your vet after the consultation, giving details of the treatment they have prescribed and any other advice concerning your dog's care that they have given. If you request a referral for your dog, your vet is usually obliged to refer you.

2 CHOOSING YOUR DOG

Dogs are our link to paradise. They don't know evil or jealousy or discontent. To sit with a dog on a hillside on a glorious afternoon is to be back in Eden, where doing nothing was not boring, it was peace.

Milan Kundera

INTRODUCTION

This chapter takes you through the important questions you need to ask yourself before getting a dog. By considering the bigger picture, and how a dog will fit in with your everyday life, as well as with your future plans, you will discover whether it would be the right choice for you. Next, having decided to get one, we will look at the factors that make dogs behave and look the way that they do, so that you can find your perfect canine match. You'll see that it is much more about nurture than it is about nature, and that it is not wise to make generalizations and assumptions about breed-specific character traits. Every dog is first and foremost an individual. This chapter also covers aspects of holistic health, through the Traditional Chinese Medicine concept of the five elements. Finally, a few tips about where to get your dog, and an introduction to some of the important legal aspects of dog ownership.

SHOULD I GET A DOG?

Every year Battersea Dogs Home alone cares for nearly 9,000 unwanted dogs, taking in, on average, twenty-three dogs every day, 365 days a year. That's why it's important to think very carefully before

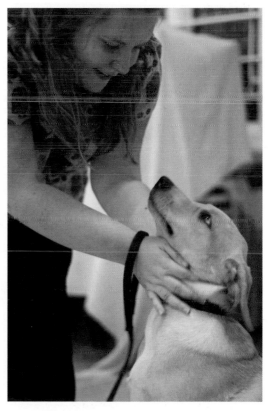

Your dog can be your best friend.

getting a dog so that you are certain that you can offer him all the care and compassion that he will need, for life. Visit friends with dogs, even ask to borrow theirs for a trial, get the feel of what it's really like to be a dog owner.

What will a dog need from me?

It pays to realize certain things about dog ownership that may not be immediately obvious. Firstly, a dog has certain important needs concerning his health and welfare, and as his owner you will be responsible for making sure that these are met. So, what are a dog's needs?

- **A home** He will need a suitable home environment, where he can feel secure, as well as warm, dry and protected.

- **Food and water** He will need a suitable diet and constant access to clean, fresh water.

- **Routine and emergency health care** Your dog will need routine preventive health care, as well as treatment if he is unwell.

- **The opportunity to mix with other dogs** He needs to get the chance to perform natural, social behaviour with his own species.

- **Regular access to the outdoors** He will need somewhere he can dig, sniff, roll around and otherwise do doggy things. This is why having a garden is usually an important prerequisite for having a dog.

- **Regular walks and the freedom to run around** Ideally, your dog should have the chance to be free, off the lead, at

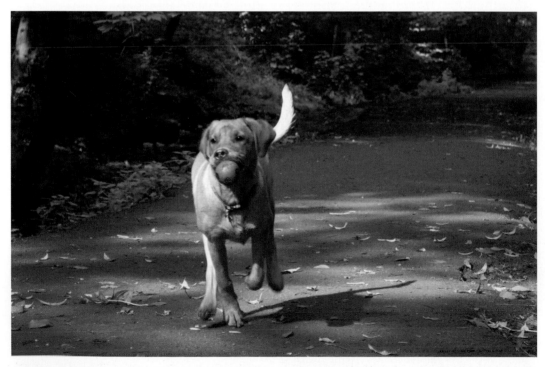

A dog will need regular walks and freedom to run around.

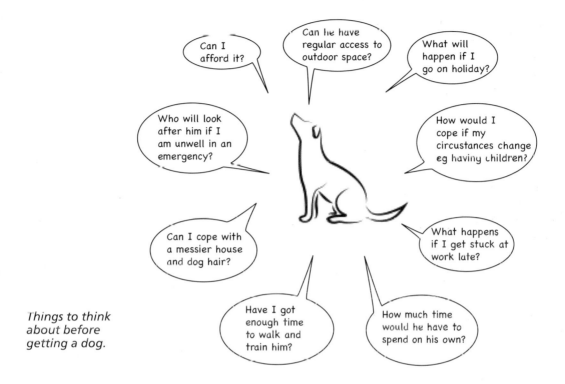

Things to think about before getting a dog.

least every few days if not more frequently.

Finally, don't forget that your dog also needs love, care and understanding. This is by no means an exhaustive list, and for sure some dogs will have more requirements than have been listed here. These are just the basics, adapted from the Animal Welfare Act 2006, which outlines the minimum requirements for acceptable dog welfare. They may sound simple and straightforward, but you need to consider whether you will be able to provide all these things for your dog on an ongoing basis, throughout his life.

Things to consider before getting a dog
There are a handful of key questions that you need to ask yourself before you can

decide whether you can provide a dog with a suitable home. Important points to remember are that it is a long-term commitment, and also that there are usually more people to consider than just yourself. How will the rest of the family cope with or respond to a dog? Who will you be relying on to look after your dog if you have an emergency or have to work late, for instance? Are you going to take your dog on holidays with you? If so, have you got realistic expectations about the limitations that this will impose on your travels? How fair would it be for your dog to have to spend long periods in kennels? Having enough time to care for a dog is another major factor. Think about how long it will take to train, exercise and care for him every day. What is his lifespan? How does this fit in with your work commitments and life plans? Are these likely to change? It's true what they say; 'A dog is for life, not just for Christmas'. In addition, make sure that you have reasonable expectations about the possible changes a dog will bring in terms of the cleanliness and tidiness of your home. If you are very house proud then this could be an issue. Cost is undeniably another key factor to consider before getting a dog, and will vary widely depending on his size, and other needs. Ongoing maintenance costs include food and routine veterinary care, and may or may not also involve regular clipping and grooming, kennels, dog-walkers and training classes. There is also the issue of being able to cover emergency treatments and illness. Pet insurance may give you peace of mind for such eventualities and many now cover the cost of complementary treatments, but make sure you always read the small print on any policy. The list of important considerations before getting a dog goes on and on, but thinking about all the possible consequences beforehand is far better than coping with unexpected problems later on.

The benefits of dog ownership

Now that you have considered all the practicalities and possible pitfalls of dog ownership, make sure you haven't forgotten why you wanted one in the first place. Here are just some of the reasons why having a dog is good for you.

- **Companionship and exercise** With around one in five people living alone in the UK, dogs can provide companionship. The daily dog walk is also an excellent way of getting regular exercise and helping you to stay fit and healthy.

- **Communication and interaction** For some people, especially the elderly, their dog may be the sole reason they have for leaving the house every day. Their dog is their only means of exercise, fresh air and the chance of having a chat with someone.

- **Health** A growing body of evidence reports that having a dog improves your health and leads to a longer and happier life. Statistics show that dog owners make fewer visits to their doctor each year, suffer fewer sleeping difficulties and are less likely to be taking medicines. It is now widely accepted that the physiological health and emotional well-being of the elderly are enhanced by contact with animals. The Ancient Greeks kept dogs in their temples; a lick from a dog was traditionally believed to be healing, and recent research proves its antibacterial properties.

- **Connection to nature and the outdoors** Walking your dog every day helps to keep you in touch with the world around you, connecting you to the weather, the seasons and your local community. This is fundamental to why having a dog is good for your health; it both grounds and connects you to the world around you.

- **Family pet** Researchers have shown that by having a dog in the family, children learn to be more nurturing, independent and responsible than those without contact with animals. Teaching your children how to behave and interact around dogs so as not to frighten them is part of a parent's responsibility. However, it is crucial to realize that no dog, however much you may know and trust him, will be 100 per cent safe with children, so don't leave them together unsupervised.

- **Guide dogs and working dogs** Dogs still play important roles as working animals. For example, they are the eyes, ears and hands of some people, and for others they are the alert system for impending epileptic fits. There are also police dogs and rescue dogs, as well as farm dogs.
- **Dogs for fun and hobbies** Training dogs for various agility sports, or to show them, are other popular reasons for having a dog. These activities are also great ways to build up mutual trust and obedience between you.
- **Friendship** Dogs are man's (and woman's) best friend – we all know that.

For all of these reasons, and more, there is growing interest, across a variety of disciplines, in the relationship between pets and health. A range of therapeutic, mind, body and spirit benefits of having

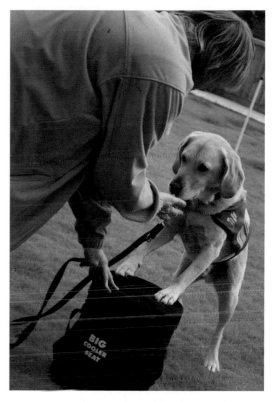

Dogs can be trained to assist people with disabilities.

pets are now well documented. The study of the human-animal bond is called Anthrozoology, and the International Association of Human-Animal Interaction recently declared that it is a universal, natural and basic human right to benefit from the presence of animals. However, it seems more ethical and respectful to consider our relationship with dogs to be a privilege, rather than a right.

CHOOSING YOUR DOG

Every dog is an individual
Every dog is different, and you can't tell what his character, temperament or

---

**PROS AND CONS OF
DOG OWNERSHIP**

Benefits
- Better health
- Exercise and fitness
- Reduces stress
- Companionship
- Meeting people
- Hobbies, e.g. dog agility

Drawbacks
- Time commitment
- Regular walks
- Regular attention
- Restrictions on spontaneous trips
- Costs
- Mud, mess and dog hair

WHAT FACTORS SHAPE YOUR DOG'S CHARACTER?

His breed However, this plays a lesser role than is usually presumed.

His genetics What your dog's mum and dad were like.

His learning experiences and environment during his socialization period This is the most important aspect of what makes your dog the way he is.

His learning experiences throughout life What your dog has seen and done, and how he has been treated.

behaviour will be like from his breed or looks alone. Getting a dog based on the assumption that he will behave a certain way because of his breed is unfortunately not possible. Just as you can't judge a book by its cover, you can't judge how a dog will behave based on what he looks like or what breed he is. We now understand the great role upbringing and learning experiences play in shaping a dog's character, making nurture rather than nature a more important factor in how he is likely to behave.

What do you want your dog to look like?

The physical attributes of the dog you choose will no doubt be important from a practical as well as an aesthetic point of view; after all, you have to enjoy looking at him. Choosing a dog that is the right size for you, and that has a type of coat you can manage, is important. It is also worth spending time considering which

sex of dog to get, and whether an adult or a puppy would be best.

Size
This is going to be one of the most obvious considerations when choosing your dog. Big dogs need more space. Easy. But size also comes into play when you think about handling and transporting him. Will you be able to restrain and cope with your dog on your own when he is full-grown and potentially very strong? Will he fit in your car comfortably? It is also true that medical bills will be higher for bigger dogs, as most medicines are prescribed based on body weight. However, while it's important to be realistic,

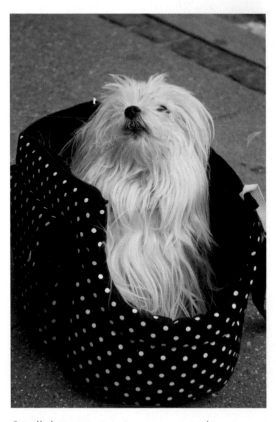

Small dogs are easy to carry around.

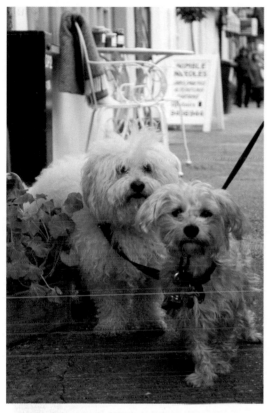

The amount of exercise a dog needs doesn't necessarily depend on his size.

also the cost of spaying to account for, which is usually higher than that of having a male neutered. Factors to consider before getting a male dog include the possibility of him going after nearby bitches on heat. It is not easy to make generalizations about differences relating to character or temperament between the sexes, as it very much depends on the individual. However, there is usually a size difference, with dogs tending to be larger than bitches.

Age

Puppy, adult, or elderly dog? The choice between getting a puppy and a mature dog encompasses a huge range of factors. Puppies will usually require a lot more time and commitment than adult dogs to begin with, and of course, taking on a puppy will be a responsibility for his whole life, which may be up to twenty years. Younger dogs are likely to need more exercise than older ones. Rescue dogs, usually taken on as adults, may come with already learnt behaviours. These may be good or bad, and in some cases they too may need a greater time commitment for retraining.

don't forget that a dog's size isn't necessarily related to how much exercise he will need; some big dogs need less exercise than small ones.

Sex

Ultimately this is going to be based on your personal choice. But remember that unless you have her spayed, a bitch will come into season twice a year. This will entail mess in the house and also means having to keep her away from male dogs during this period. Otherwise, if she did get pregnant and have puppies, you would have to deal with this too. There is

Coat type

Do you choose a long- or a shorthaired dog? Did you realize that many breeds have to be taken to the groomers regularly to have their coats clipped or hand stripped? Do you have the time to brush your dog's coat every day? For many longhaired breeds this is a necessity. Equally, if you are deep in the countryside where getting wet and muddy will be a daily occurrence, will a longhaired dog be too 'high maintenance'? Are you allergic to dog hair? In which case choosing a breed such as a poodle, which is non-shedding, will be important.

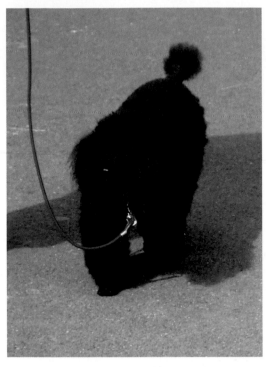

Poodles don't moult and so may be good for people with allergies.

PEDIGREE OR MIXED BREED?

This section highlights the main reasons for choosing a pedigree dog or a mixed breed, or whether you should consider adopting a rescue dog. Knowing the key issues relating to each will help you to make an informed decision about the best kind of dog for you.

A short history of dog breeds

Until the late nineteenth century dogs were selectively bred for their working abilities and traits that were helpful for their function in life. In those days dogs had all kinds of jobs, from hunting to pulling carts, herding sheep, and protecting farms. The individuals that had the best abilities would have been selectively bred, so that the breeds became even cleverer and more skilled. However, just over two hundred years ago the priorities in dog breeding changed. There was less need for working dogs, and kennel clubs, breed societies and dog showing started to take off, so that breeding for appearance, instead of function, began. Nowadays we have a huge variation in the physical appearances of our dogs, from the Chihuahua to the Great Dane. This is why it is sometimes easy to fall into the trap of basing their identities on their breed, rather than on the fact that they are all part of the same species – the dog.

Pedigrees

A pedigree, or pure breed dog, is one that has been selectively bred to show particular characteristics and to look a certain way. If he has his ancestry and lineage recorded (usually through the Kennel Club), he will be designated a 'pedigree dog'. This refers to the fact that there is a written record of his breeding. In most cases you are more likely to be considering the 'pedigree' question if you are getting a puppy. However, with rehoming centres and welfare schemes for most breeds, you can also get pedigree dogs 'second hand', as rescues. Getting a dog of a certain breed, with a known family background, is certainly an excellent predictor of how he will look. However, do remember that it is not a good predictor of how he will behave. While it is true that we may have selectively bred for certain traits in dogs of certain breeds, such as increased responsiveness in collies and perseverance in terriers, how these traits are expressed depends on the individual dog. It relates to what the dog has learnt throughout his life and what his past experiences have been. It is simply impossible to generalize about individual dogs based on their breed. Unfortunately, it is this common misconception that dogs will be more likely to behave in a particular way based on how they look that has led to so many dogs arriving at Battersea Dogs Home. They simply didn't behave as they were expected to for their breed. Other reasons for choosing a pedigree are linked to the familiarity of having had, and loved, that type of dog before, in childhood for example. Another factor associated with pedigree dogs is that of status. Dogs of certain breeds can undeniably provoke certain assumptions about the owner and their lifestyle and hence their social status. It pays to be honest with yourself about why you like a particular breed of dog, and whether his needs, not just his looks, fit your lifestyle and how you can provide for him. 'Status dogs' are not a new phenomenon; dogs have been status symbols for as long as man has needed to show he is better than his neighbour. Roman Emperors bred Salukis and would take their biggest and best ones out into battle with them, and even had mosaics of dogs on the entrance gates of their villas. Chinese statesmen bred the Pekingese especially small to be able to fit into the sleeves of their robes, a sign of nobility and high state. Nowadays there are still clear trends associated with the popularity of certain breeds. Recently there has been a huge increase in the popularity of fighting dogs, or dogs used for intimidation, such as the Staffordshire Bull Terrier.

Form over function

Unfortunately, breeding for looks has taken its toll on the calibre of certain breeds. These dogs have been selectively

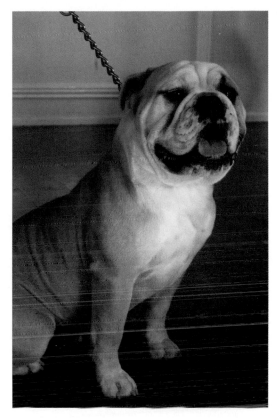

Pedigree dogs have been selectively bred.

bred with an emphasis on extreme physical features at the expense of their health and welfare. It's simple really: you just have to look at some of these dogs, the Bulldog or the Shar-pei for instance, to appreciate that they can't live normal, healthy lives when they look the way they do. You don't have to be a vet to see that the Pug, with its very compressed muzzle, will have trouble breathing, or that the Bassett, with its ears that drag on the ground and its heavy body and small legs, will be susceptible to ear infections and early onset arthritis. It is sad that these 'abnormalities' have come to be called 'attributes'. The fact is that these unique and individualizing features, which once made the breed stand out, have been exaggerated too much. This has been done so that these dogs can conform to kennel clubs' 'breed standards' and so win prizes. A short nose or long ears are fine, and indeed may have originally been beneficial to the dog's work or role, in hounds for instance, but only up to a point. This limit has obviously been breached with several breeds now struggling with the everyday functions of life, such as walking and breathing. By restricting the number of individuals that are allowed to produce offspring, the gene pools of certain breeds have also become severely limited. This increases the risks of inherited diseases for certain breeds, such as hip dysplasia, epilepsy and heart disease. So, when choosing a pedigree dog, as well as making sure that common sense tells you he won't suffer because of how he looks, also bear in mind the possibility of inherited medical problems that won't be obvious from the outside. Do your homework and find out the inherited diseases or complaints to which your chosen breed may be susceptible and whether there are any screening programmes in place to check for them. Fundamentally, the best thing that you can do to help stop this unsound practice of selective breeding for aesthetics at the expense of animal welfare is not to buy into it. There are many breeds that are not 'extreme' in their looks, and hence will be healthy, happy dogs. Use your

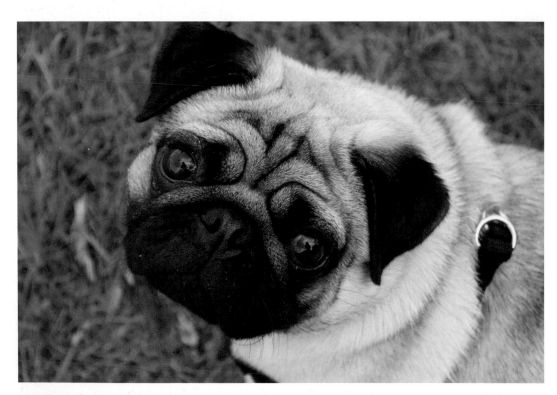

The Pug's lovable features can sometimes make it difficult for him to breathe.

common sense and do your research. It is time for a new era of dog breeding, one based on a full understanding of canine biology, that values health, longevity and a suitable temperament over looks alone.

Screening for inherited conditions in pedigree dogs

Many medical conditions have a genetic component to them. Therefore, to help reduce the incidence of such conditions, reputable breeders test their dogs before they are bred from to make sure they are not likely to pass any known condition to their offspring. So, before getting a pedigree dog, have a word with your vet to see what specific screening tests are available for the particular breed you are considering. The results of these tests should be included in the registration documents for your puppy. It is not only physical characteristics that are inherited; temperament problems are also passed from parent to offspring. This is why it is so important that you meet the parents, or at least the mother, of your prospective puppy.

Mixed breeds

Most dogs are a mix of two or more breeds, and will have an ancestry that, beyond the parents at least, is generally unknown. It is widely believed that these mixed-breed dogs, also known as mongrels, are healthier than their pedigree cousins thanks to their 'hybrid vigour'. They are also less likely to suffer from inherited conditions due to their more varied genetic make-up. While you may be able to guess the eventual adult size of a mixed-breed puppy by what he looks like and what breeds he is made up of, this will not help you assess his future temperament. His past learning experiences and what has happened to him throughout his life will govern this, and so will often be a complete unknown. Choosing a mixed-breed dog often means that you are taking on a rescue dog, or one that is unwanted or has been abandoned. This is of course a better ethical and 'green' choice than getting a specially bred puppy, and is increasingly popular with socially responsible owners who believe in recycling! It can be argued that another reason for choosing a rescue or mixed-breed dog is that it has a lower environmental impact, or carbon 'paw print', than the less sustainable pedigree. It also means that your dog will be absolutely unique and one of a kind.

It is worth noting that a 'crossbreed' dog is a cross between two pedigree breeds, rather than having the more varied make-up of the 'mixed breed'. Crossbreeds are becoming increasingly trendy, with new combinations emerging all the time. For example, the Cockapoo (a Cocker Spaniel/Poodle cross) and the Labradoodle (Labrador/Poodle cross).

THE RESCUE DOG

Getting a rescue dog can be much more of a gamble than opting for a 'new' puppy. While it can be very rewarding to give a home to an unwanted animal, you are also inheriting a dog with behaviour traits that may need patience and training to change. However, this doesn't necessarily mean that you are taking on a 'problem'; some dogs need rehoming due to their owners moving house, becoming allergic to them, or having a baby. Getting a rescue may mean, therefore, that you are taking on a well-socialized dog that has had positive learning experiences in the past, and hence is 'easy'. However, in many other cases, sadly, it means the opposite, and rescue dogs do

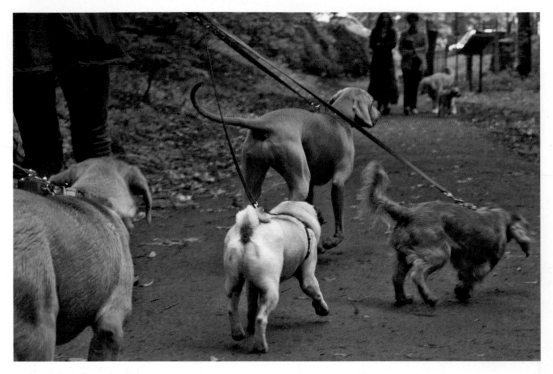

You could use a dog walker if you can't walk your dog yourself.

come with 'problems'. This is why they are frequently taken on by experienced owners, or those that are prepared for the likely extra commitment and patience.

Complementary remedies for the rescue dog

A dog from a rescue centre will usually have been through a lot of emotional upset and trauma. He will not only have lost his old 'family' but is likely to have had to spend time in a stressful, noisy kennel environment before you found him. The following Bach Flower Remedies can be very useful for helping him to recover and settle into his new home (for directions on how to administer them *see* Chapter 1).

Star of Bethlehem, for the after-effects of shock.
Rock Rose, for terror.
Sweet Chestnut, for loss and grief.
Aspen and **Mimulus**, for fears.

The homeopathic remedy for extreme grief and loss, Ignatia, can also be helpful for the rescue dog, particularly if his previous owner died, or if he has had to be separated from another dog that was his close companion. However, if your new rescue companion was in the rescue centre long-term, and appears depressed and withdrawn, the remedy called Natrum Mur is often more useful. Both of these can be used at a potency (strength) of 200c twice daily for a maximum of two days.

THE FIVE ELEMENTS AND HOLISTIC HEALTH CARE

By turning to the Traditional Chinese Medicine (TCM) five element theory, we can gain further insight into the general health of your dog. Based on his unique constitutional characteristics, it can be used to help predict his susceptibility to disease. According to the ancient Chinese, each of the five elements that make up the universe – fire, earth, metal, water and wood – are reflected in everything in it, including people and animals. The five element theory is used to chart patterns of health and disease, with health seen as a balance between the elements. TCM practitioners use the five element theory for diagnosis and treatment of their patients, using acupuncture and herbs to restore balance and health. Each individual can be assigned to one, or more often a combination, of the five elements. Understanding which element or elements are reflected in your dog can give you an insight into which conditions are likely to affect him, and hence what to avoid. The five element theory is a complex and integral part of TCM and takes years of study to fully understand. The following is just a snapshot, to give you a glimpse into another way of understanding health and disease.

The Fire Constitution

These are anxious, hyperactive, high-energy dogs that have a tendency towards hysteria, often barking and yapping. They thrive on fuss and attention and can suffer from separation anxiety if left on their own. They can also be prone to heart and circulatory disorders, as the Chinese Medicine organs associated with 'fire' are the heart and its protective case, the pericardium. These dogs are likely to be uncomfortable in the heat, with any complaints they suffer from being worse in the summer.

The Earth Constitution

These are stocky, well-built dogs that are generally loyal, routine-loving individuals, with a tendency to worry. 'Earth' type dogs are always willing to please and are extremely sensitive to their owner's moods. This element is linked to the digestive system, hence the tendency towards becoming overweight and to suffer from conditions such as diarrhoea or colitis. Their ailments tend to be aggravated by damp weather and by any change to their routine.

The Metal Constitution

This element is often linked to dogs that are slim and delicate in their build. These individuals will have a slightly melancholy, sad air about them, as the emotion associated with this element is grief. Therefore these metal-type dogs will be particularly badly affected by events such as the loss of their owner, or rehoming. This element is linked to the respiratory system, so there is a tendency for these dogs to suffer from ailments such as colds, coughs, or asthma. They suffer most ailments in the autumn, as it is dry and cold conditions that are detrimental to the metal constitution.

The Water Constitution

Water-type dogs have a tendency to be anxious; they can appear aggressive, but this will be based on a feeling of fear. The sound that a water-type dog typically uses to communicate is a groan or a growl, whereas a fire type would bark, and an earth dog would sigh. Water types are susceptible to bladder or urinary tract conditions, including kidney disease. The body tissue that is linked to the water element is bone; therefore these dogs tend to suffer with arthritic complaints, especially in the lower back. Water types are affected by cold weather, especially suffering in the winter months.

The Wood Constitution

These are typically wiry, athletic dogs that have a tendency to be tense and anxious. Their bark is loud and ferocious and they can be moody and possessive over food or other resources that they value. This is because the emotions linked to the wood element are anger and frustration. Wood-type dogs tend to suffer with eye complaints, as well as from skin and nail problems. They are also susceptible to ligament and tendon strains. The weather that most aggravates wood types is the wind, and the season when they are most likely to be affected by an ailment is in the spring.

WHAT IS A PUPPY FARM?

It is like a factory farm for puppies, where dogs are bred in distressing circumstances, in very poor conditions. Bitches frequently have too many litters, and puppies are weaned too early. Such puppies can be at greater risk of inherited diseases due to inbreeding, as well as to infections due to overcrowding and stress. Farmed puppies are commonly sold to pet shops, but are also bought by dealers who then advertise them in newspapers and may masquerade as breeders themselves. These puppies may well come with a pedigree certificate. Some people feel that they have to 'rescue' them, however in reality this will unfortunately be simply supporting the trade. In order to help bring an end to puppy farming, it is crucial that you don't buy into it.

WHERE TO GET YOUR DOG

Word of mouth, or friends of friends, is generally one of the most successful ways of finding your new companion. Adverts in local vet clinics are also useful, as dogs that need new homes, as well as local puppies, are often advertised in this way. However, do be wary of getting a puppy through a newspaper or Internet advert, or from some pet shops, as according to several animal welfare association surveys, many of these will have come from puppy farms.

If you are looking to rehome a dog, rescue centres such as Battersea Dogs Home and The Dogs Trust, and all the smaller, similar organizations are usually a very good place to start. Most reputable organizations will have a rigorous process of compatibility checking to make sure that you end up with the right dog. Every dog should also have had a thorough medical check, and most will also have been neutered and microchipped before you take them home. There will usually be a nominal rehoming charge, to cover these costs as well as being an acknowledgment of taking on the responsibility of caring for your new dog. If you are looking for a dog or puppy of a particular breed then contacting the breed rescue associations is a good idea. Most breed clubs, and certainly those for the most common breeds, will have a rehoming facility.

Pedigree dogs are usually taken on as puppies. A lot of good breeders will not advertise in newspapers, instead relying on word of mouth and through links to their breed club. Some will even have waiting lists for their puppies. You should expect to get the third degree when you contact a good breeder, as they will want the best for their puppies and will need to feel sure that you can provide a good home for them. However, you can in turn ask them a lot of questions yourself, most importantly about any health screening tests that they have done. You should expect to go and collect your puppy from the breeder's house and to see the mother, your puppy and his siblings. Conscientious breeders won't mind you visiting and asking to have a look around.

RESPONSIBLE DOG OWNERSHIP

As a responsible dog owner you need to be aware of a few of the major legislations and codes of conduct that could affect you. Firstly, according to the Control of Dogs Order 1992, whenever your dog is out and about in a public place he must be wearing a collar with a tag with your name, address, postcode and telephone number on it. It is also a legal requirement for your dog to be on a lead whenever he is walked beside a road, and for you to pick up after him if he defecates in a public place. In addition, it is sensible to make sure that your dog is covered by insurance in case he is involved in an accident resulting in third party liability claims. The Animal Welfare Act 2006 lays out the expected minimum standards for dog care, and is a legal safeguard against animal cruelty. You should also know that stray dogs are collected and taken to the local council's dog wardens' offices, and not to the police.

The future for legislation

The law regarding dog ownership is due to change, with new legislation proposed

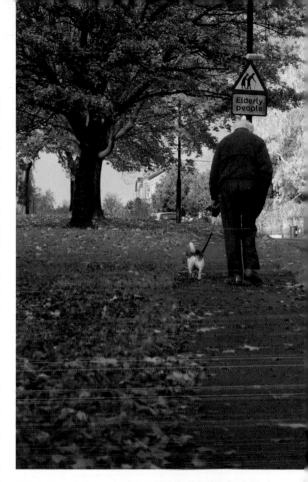

Having a dog provides companionship and regular exercise.

to replace the 1991 Dangerous Dogs Act. It is hoped that this new 'Dog Control Bill' will place the emphasis on responsible dog ownership, rather than on penalizing any particular breeds of dog. It is widely supported by dog welfare groups as well as the veterinary profession. Dog licensing is another issue that is currently being debated in parliament, and is closely linked to the call by all the major dog welfare organizations in the UK for compulsory microchipping. Making every dog traceable to his owner will help tackle the rising problem of abandoned dogs. Last year alone 97,000 dogs were found as strays, with the RSPCA taking calls about abandoned dogs every hour. The bottom line is that educating the public about 'responsible dog ownership' has to be the cornerstone for any new legislation.

Tail docking

Tail docking has been banned in England since 2007. Sadly, however, there are still exemptions to this, with certain breeds of working dog still legally allowed to have their tails docked if they can be shown to be going to working homes. Most of the veterinary profession agree that this is a mutilation that should be fully banned. All dogs need their tails for balance and communication, and docking can cause chronic pain. If you are looking for a puppy as a pet, there is no reason why you should be offered one with a docked tail.

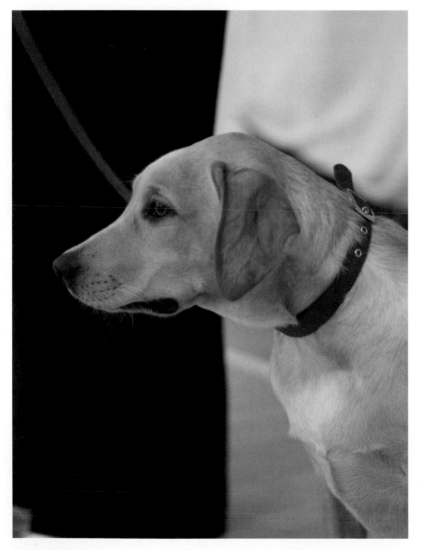

Responsible dog ownership.

3 THE CANINE MIND

Understanding basic canine psychology will give you a better appreciation of what motivates your dog and what makes him content and happy. By gaining an insight into your dog's view of the world and an appreciation of how he communicates, you will benefit from a better relationship with him.

A NEW VISION FOR UNDERSTANDING DOGS

For the past thirty years the popular model for understanding dog behaviour has been based on the concepts of pack leader, hierarchy and dominance. The need for the owner to be 'pack leader'

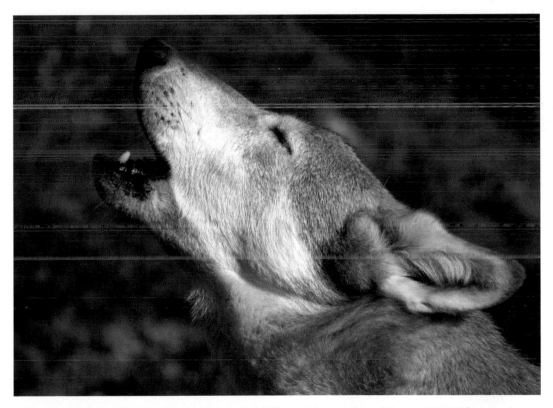

We now understand that dogs behave very differently to wolves. (Photo: UK Wolf Conservation Trust)

and show their dog that he is always subordinate has been the mainstay of every popular training method. These ideas include going through the door before your dog, never letting him eat before you, and at its most extreme involves physically forcing him to submit to you. These methods go further than just common sense and good manners and are aimed at demonstrating to your dog that you are 'top' of the pack. However, it has now been proved beyond question that these ideas and training techniques are completely outdated and ineffective. In the past ten to fifteen years, up-to-date research has given us a new understanding of how dogs live and what motivates them. We now understand that the wolf behaviour on which these dominance hierarchy ideas were based was flawed and that dogs behave very differently to wolves.

Because they are their closest ancestors, we used to believe that dogs would behave a lot like wolves. So when captive wolves were studied in the 1960s and the seminal paper outlining their behaviour was published, this was taken as gospel for wolf, and hence dog, natural behaviour. These captive wolves were very fierce, fought to gain status and rank, and had a clear hierarchy in their group, which is where today's popular, but now outdated, model comes from. These hand-reared wolves were actually an artificial pack of unrelated individuals living in captivity, which meant that they were behaving in a very unnatural way. This group should not have been a model for wolf, let alone domestic dog, behaviour. Under these conditions any animals forced to live together in a confined space would naturally compete with one another. Later, by living with and studying wolves in the wild, it was realized

that in fact they lived and behaved very differently to the captive, unrelated pack. In the wild, wolves live in small, stable, family groups where there is little aggression and certainly not a rigid hierarchy or pack leader. Their behaviour is based on cohesion and cooperation, not conflict. Moreover, even the term 'alpha pair' was shown to be invalid; although there is a breeding pair, they do not show any dominance in how they live within the pack. By this stage, when the mistake in understanding was realized in the late 1990s, the terminology and ideas of the dominant alpha dog had been too widely taken on by the public and by leading figures in the dog world for them to be changed. It is said that it takes twenty years for new scientific ideas to become generally accepted. So, although this new vision is practised by all well-regarded behaviour experts and trainers today, it is only recently that it has started to filter down to the more grass roots level of the dog-loving public.

The second reason that this theory is outdated is because comparing dog behaviour to that of the wolf is not as helpful as was first thought. Although they share a common ancestor, hundreds of years of domestication have altered the dog and made him into a completely different species to the wolf. Even though they do still have some similar, innate 'wolf-like' behaviour patterns, we should also see that dogs are very different animals, domestic as opposed to wild.

One interesting way of looking at the changing view of dog behaviour theory is to see it reflected in the models by which the human population lives and works. The system of hierarchy, rank, and dominance that we saw in our dogs matched the predominant human social structure in the workplace during the 70s and 80s.

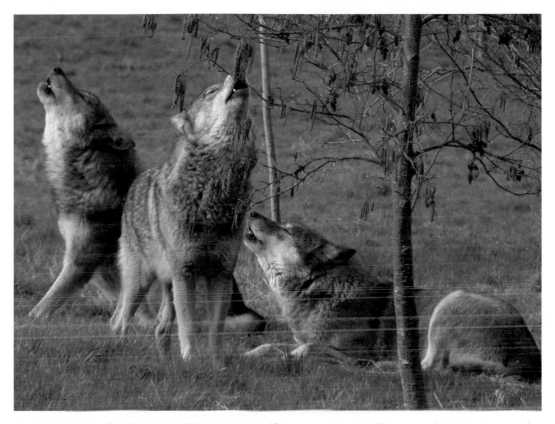

A wolf pack is a family group. (Photo: UK Wolf Conservation Trust)

But now, as we are moving towards a more fluid, less hierarchical, way of living and working ourselves, we are starting to alter the way we treat and understand our dogs, to reflect this.

To get a fuller appreciation of what makes our dogs tick, and hence how best to interact and train them, we will investigate how dogs communicate, what happens when we misunderstand them and the importance of socialization and training. First we will take a more detailed look at wolf behaviour, and also that of feral dog packs. This will illustrate the difference between the behaviour of wild animals and those captive animals involved in the outdated behavioural studies.

The wolf

A wolf pack is a family group, with a mum and dad and various offspring, from pups to two-year-olds. The parents or elder siblings guide, teach and protect the youngsters. All members of the group communicate with each other in order to live in harmony, hunt effectively, reduce injury and rear pups successfully. They are not dominating other members of the pack, and there is no constant struggle over pecking order. For example, if there is not much food available for the pack then the pups will always eat first. The only time there is the potential for conflict, and a struggle for position within the pack, is between older siblings. For example, between brothers of the same age and size there may be some fighting to try and find their position in order to live together. In these cases, this will be the time when one or both animals start going out to find their own pack and territory.

The domestic dog

Domestication was the process whereby wolves were selectively bred over generations to become the friendly, sociable animals that we can share our homes with today, the domestic dog (*canis familiaris*).

As well as breeding from the most docile and sociable individuals, domestication also involved selectively breeding for adults with puppy-like characteristics. This is because puppies are more adaptable and easier to train and control than adults, so can become more readily accustomed to humans. Hence, selectively breeding adult animals to stay as puppy-like as possible was of benefit to early man. These puppy-like qualities included being physically smaller and having bigger ears and a high-pitched bark, as well as being mentally more adaptable, playful and eager to please. Knowing this is important for understanding how our dogs behave and hence how we should reasonably treat them.

Although they are descended from the wolf, today's domestic dog is a completely different species and their behaviours bear much less resemblance to each other than was previously believed. Instead of comparing dog behaviour to that of the wolf, we can get a much better insight by examining how feral dogs live and behave. Feral dogs are domestic dogs whose behaviour isn't influenced by people, and so they are a much better model for comparison than wolves. Indeed, as opposed to wolves, feral dogs have very little need to operate as a true pack. They live as small groups surviving by scavenging for food, and are far less family-oriented than wolves, having less need to communicate with one another since they are not working together to hunt. Feral dogs are rarely seen using cooperative behaviour, and indeed often live on their own. Overall it seems that domestication has radically changed the social behaviour of dogs, so that when they have the chance to interact and breed freely, as they do in feral groups, they live in very loose associations that are not as family-oriented and close-knit as that of the wolf.

However, as well as domesticating them, we have also bred dogs selectively over generations for specific purposes such as herding, guarding and hunting. Therefore it must not be forgotten that their emotional health and balance will depend upon their being able to fulfil, or at least have an activity that mimics, these innate desires and tasks. This could be in the way that you play with your dog, the kinds of walks you provide, or the agility or training classes you take him to, or indeed the toys that he has. Of course this desire and drive will vary between individuals, but it is true to say that in some dogs the original working temperament will be strong.

HOW DOGS COMMUNICATE

We may think it's easy to understand what our dog is saying to us: when they tap their bowl they want feeding, when they bring us their lead it's time for a

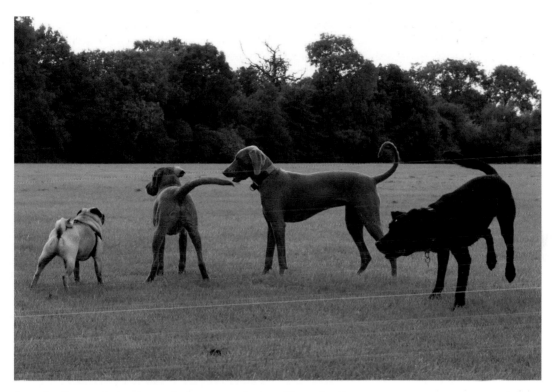

Dogs' tails are vital to how they communicate with each other.

walk. However, when the situation is less clear-cut and the signals are more subtle, then it is easy to misinterpret them. Don't forget we speak different languages, and just as you would put in time and effort to learn French or German, for example, it is important to expend a little effort learning to read and speak 'dog'. This means observing your dog and seeing how he reacts in different situations, and what his likes and dislikes are. Watch his body posture, how his ears are positioned, his lips and mouth, his eyes, his hackles, the position of his tail (all explained below). Don't just observe these things in your own dog, remember to practise your observational skills by carefully watching every dog you see and meet. Just as with any new language, take every chance you have to practise. Become aware of how your dog acts in a variety of different situations, such as at home or somewhere new, a friend's house or a potentially scary place such as the vet's. Observe how he greets new dogs on a walk or in the park, when he is both on and off the lead. Quietly watching him, without interacting, will be the best way of gaining an understanding of what makes him tick and hence learning to hear and understand what it is that he is trying to tell you. Again, it is easy to give a human interpretation to the signals that your dog is showing you; this is a trap that many owners fall into. Such misinterpretation should be avoided at all costs because it affects the way that you respond and react to your dog. If you have read the situation incorrectly and have attached the wrong human emotion to your dog's responses, then you may inadvertently be reinforcing fearfulness, for example. The best way to avoid getting things wrong is to keep things simple and just look at what your dog is doing, and the context he is doing it in. Then try and put yourself into his shoes and see the situation from his point of view as a dog, not a person. This is obviously complicated. The main idea to take away from here is to work on your 'dog language' skills of 'listening' and 'seeing', and then if necessary consult an expert for the interpretation. In other words, be cautious about humanizing what you think you see your dog doing. It is far better to seek expert advice to check that you understand the situation completely, than risk misinterpreting it and potentially making it worse. This will take time; just as you don't fully understand a potential friend or partner in the first five minutes, or pick up a new language after one lesson, it will be an ongoing learning curve.

Body language

Your dog may try and tell you how he is feeling through his body position, his facial expression and his actions. However, unless you are observant it is easy to miss these signals or even to misinterpret them. Your dog's body language will also be a product of his previous learning experiences – what signals and body positions he has learnt to do in order to get certain responses. But, as a general rule, an upright posture, where your dog attempts to make himself bigger by rais-

ing his hackles, with head held high and ears and tail erect, are signs that he is on the alert and ready for action. Conversely, if he is cowering and crouching down and making himself small, ears flat to his head, licking his lips, or yawning, your dog is signalling that he is anxious. Tail wagging is just a signal that your dog is ready to react. It could mean that he is happy and excited; however, it could also mean that he is fearful, it all depends on the context in which he is doing it. A fearful dog tucks his tail between his legs and holds his head down, avoids eye contact and may even show a grin-like expression by pulling his lips back. At its extreme he may roll over and show his tummy as a sign of appeasement, just as he may do when he's happy. We can also recognize the 'play bow', where the dog lowers his fore-limbs while keeping his bottom in the air; this is a posture that says I want to play, I'm not looking for a fight. These are the kinds of visual signals that well-socialized dogs will use to tell other dogs what is going on and how they are feeling. This usually allows them to avoid conflict by being able to size one another up from a long way off. Body posture and body position are thus crucial in inter-dog communication. Just as it is now realized that there is no hierarchical system between man and dog, the same is true between dogs. That is to say, when dogs either live together within a household, or meet in the park, becoming dominant or 'top of the pack' is not an issue. They just want to check each other out, just as we are curious when we meet someone new. Then they will either play or chase, or move along and get on with the walk if the other dog seems uninteresting.

Long before a dog will bite or snap at you, he will usually have shown a whole range of signs to try and tell you, in dog-language, that he feels threatened and wants you to back off. If none of these messages gets through to you, and you continue to do something that makes him anxious or unhappy, he is left with his final resort, his teeth. It may sometimes seem that a dog has gone straight for the biting option. However, this is rarely the case and would only have become a pattern of behaviour if you, or his previous owners, had repeatedly missed his signals of anxiety. Hence he no longer uses these any more but goes straight for the one that is always understood, the bite. Dogs that have reached this point and have actually bitten people need professional help from qualified behaviourists.

Appearance

It isn't just humans that misinterpret the signs. Dogs too are often very bad at communicating with each other. This is due to poor socialization as puppies, the way that they have been bred to look, and also, inadvertently, how we have trained them.

Some pedigree breeds have such extreme variations on normal anatomy that it is hard or impossible for another dog to tell whether they are friendly or anxious. This is quite simply because selective breeding has resulted in dogs with short, squashed-up noses, staring eyes, wrinkled skin, floppy ears and short or docked tails. These individuals, for example the Pekingese or the Cavalier King Charles Spaniel, with their promi-

These dogs are using their tails for balance as well as communication.

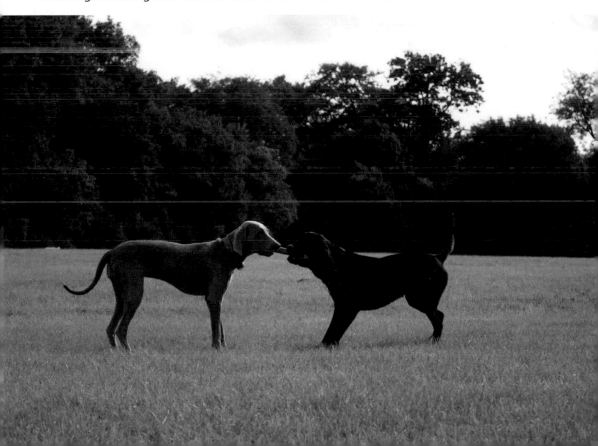

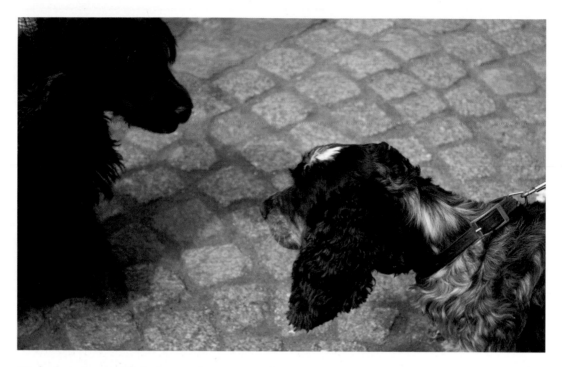

These two dogs are gently greeting one another.

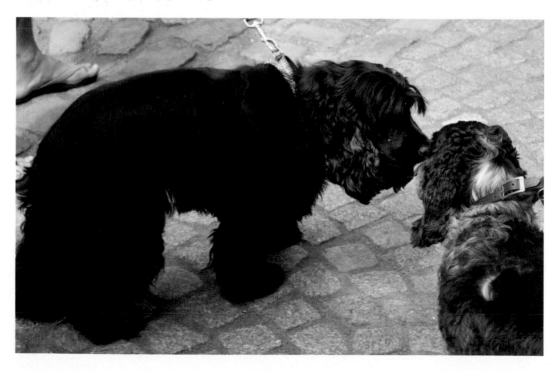

nent eyes, cannot communicate properly with other dogs. Their man-manipulated bodies can give out provocative signals. Equally the docking of tails has removed another of their signals for alerting other dogs that they are friendly, or in a bad mood. Studies carried out at the University of Southampton have shown that the range of so-called submissive and aggressive behaviours shown by a breed is closely related to their physical appearance.

Dogs communicate using all their senses: sight, smell, sound, taste and touch. This is why we need to be aware of how they use each of these in order to interpret what they are trying to tell us, as well as how they are feeling towards other dogs. The visual signals they use are unique in that they include facial expressions. Dogs are one of the few mammals, apart from humans, to do this. This is why the excessive facial folds of breeds such as the Shar-Pei, and also the very squashed-up noses and flattened faces of some other breeds, are such a hindrance to how they communicate. Indeed, fascinating new research has shown that dogs are capable of picking up on very subtle changes in facial expressions. However, don't expect this to be as easy the other way round. Your dog's facial expressions may not mean what you take them to mean; for example, the lips going back into a grin is a sign of anxiety, rather being the friendly smile of the human social repertoire. Your dog's signals and signs are subtle and complex, and for you to have the best chance of interpreting them correctly they need to be considered in context, according to the circumstances and situation.

Smell

With bottom sniffing being such an everyday greeting between dogs, it's not easy to forget that smell is one of the most crucial ways that dogs exchange information about one another. The scent produced by the anal glands

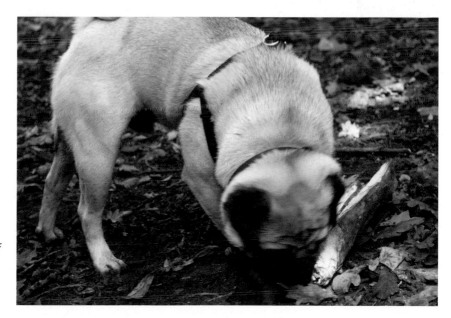

A dog's sense of smell is many hundreds of times greater than ours.

provides a whole history unique to the individual dog. By sniffing one another's bottoms, dogs can exchange information about how old they are, their sexual state, where they live, where they have been, what their mood is and probably lots more. The smell sensor area of their brains is much larger than that of sight, so that dogs can detect odours at concentrations many hundreds of times lower than we can. As well as directly smelling other dog's bottoms, they will usually also have a good sniff at the scent marks left in the urine or faeces of other dogs. Here they will get all the similar information about the other dog. These scents are also markers for territory.

Sound

The range of what dogs can communicate to each other audibly is vast, and many different sounds have been identified, from a whimper to a bark, each having a different quality and a particular tone. However, always interpret the sounds that your dog makes in relation to the context in which he is making them. The growl can be a defence warning, but also a play signal, and the whine can mean anything from a sign of pain to an attention-seeking call. It is his past learning experiences that help to inform the way that your dog chooses to use certain vocalizations in particular circumstances. This is why it can be different in every dog. You can't necessarily tell from the sound that your dog is making what he is trying to tell you; you have to look at his body language and the circumstances too.

Puppy traits

There is no denying the fact that through domestication and the selection for juvenile characteristics, we have bred dogs to retain childish behaviour into adulthood.

Thus they have ended up with puppy or adolescent behaviours and physical features. If this selective breeding had not been adopted, then family dogs today would have a more independent personality and might be more difficult to train and include in everyday life. Importantly, even with this breeding the modern dog can still make a very good parent to its young.

In summary

It is clear that your dog will try and communicate with you just as he would with another dog. This is most obviously demonstrated to you by his posture and body signals, ears up or down, lips drawn back or mouth open, and the sounds he makes, from a growl to a whimper. Therefore, by being aware that he is using all these ways of 'talking' to you and 'telling' you how he is feeling, you should be better placed to understand your dog and live happily together, as a two-species family.

HOW WE INFLUENCE OUR PETS

The holistic perspective

It's no coincidence that people are like their pets in more than just looks. Calm, patient, gentle owners seem to have the same qualities reflected in the behaviour of their dogs. In contrast, people who are highly-strung, stressed and anxious tend to have dogs that are more on edge and wary. This is partly of course because we tend to pick dogs with whom we feel an affinity; so if you are an anxious, nervous type, you may well be drawn to animals that also exhibit these qualities. However, the other reason for the similarities lies in a shared energy, one consequence of which is the phenomenon of mirror-neurones. People who live together tend to reflect one another's actions; parents often comment on it when they see their own gestures, way of walking, or facial expression copied by their baby. The same goes for family pets mirroring the way that they experience their owner's behaviour and reaction patterns.

The other consequence of shared energy between our dogs and us is that they tend to soak up our negative energies, such as sadness, anxieties and frustrations. According to holistic medical philosophies, in which the mind and body are parts of a dynamic whole, these emotions, when prolonged or very strong, can actually lead to physical ailments. In Traditional Chinese Medicine fear links to the kidneys, anger to the liver and grief to the lungs (the five elements and the correspondences). Coupled with the belief, fundamental to holistic medicine, that energy (qi or vital force) is the source of all processes and functions that keep us alive, this allows us to appreciate how prolonged negative emotional states can affect physical health. This may well explain why we see illnesses shared between owners and their pets (epilepsy, cancer and diabetes, for example). Even if you don't believe in qi, or shared energy, it has been demonstrated that stress-related ailments in pets could be linked to their owner's emotional state. Therefore, it pays to be aware of how our moods and way of reacting affect the way our dogs behave, and even their health. Reducing the potential for transferring your negative emotions onto your dog may be an idea that you want to take on board. For example, if you have had a particularly tough day at the office and feel angry and frustrated, give yourself a little 'time out' to process your feelings in another way, a walk or a run for instance, before rushing in to cuddle your

dog. By doing this, you will possibly have less negative energy to share with your dog. Indeed, on another level, it may mean that you will also have less potential for being impatient or cross with him. Hence it will also be advantageous for your dog's training and learning.

SOCIALIZATION

The importance of early life

The earliest part of a puppy's life, from when they open their eyes at about three weeks until they are about six months old, is crucially important to what sort of dog they will become in later life. In other words, the foundations of a well-rounded and balanced adult dog are laid down in these first few months. This is because during this period puppies are naturally curious about, rather than scared of, new things and can therefore learn that they are harmless and fine. If the young dog encounters new objects after this 'critical period' between roughly three and twelve weeks of age, then his natural reaction is to be wary and fearful. By exposing him to literally as much as you can in these crucial early stages, you can make sure that you are laying the foundations for a 'bomb proof' dog. However, it is very important that these interactions and new experiences are positive, and that they are controlled. This means that your puppy is never overwhelmed or frightened by the new things. For example, it's a great idea to get him used to the loud bangs and screams of fireworks, but do this at some distance and only for a short time. Don't go and stand with him at the very front in a big fireworks display, as this will set him up for being scared of them for life. Studies comparing dogs that were brought up in different environments

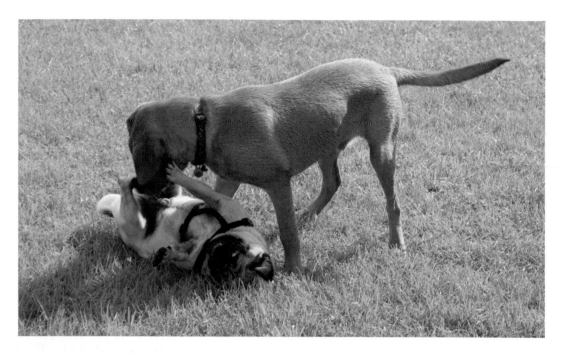

Play is a valuable learning experience for dogs.

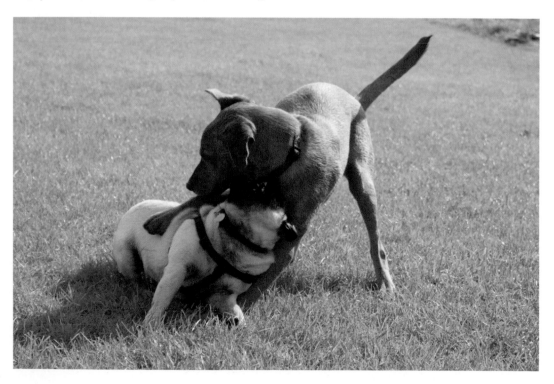

repeatedly confirm that giving them a rich social life and a stimulating physical environment during their first six months is associated with a reduced incidence of behaviour problems later on. This is supported by the fact that we now know that it is much more 'nurture' than 'nature' that makes people into the adults they become. It has very little to do with genes, and is much more linked to our early care and how our parents treated us. Having a well-behaved dog that does what he is told, comes back when he is called, and can walk on the lead, is not only beneficial for us, but it makes life for the dog a much happier existence. It's not a myth that dogs thrive on routine and knowing what to expect; this is the basis for a contented, confident and happy dog.

GOOD BEHAVIOUR

Think positive

Just as your thoughts and ideas will inform your own actions, it's all about thinking positive when you are training your dog. If you want good behaviour and a well-trained and responsive dog, then carry a mental picture of that sort of dog in your mind. Of course this isn't all there is to it. You will still need to actually do the training and go to the classes, but having the right mental framework in place to help you achieve your aims is a powerful tool. Have a mental picture of your dog coming back when you call him or lying calmly at your feet and sitting unfazed in his basket when the doorbell rings. Try to focus only on positive images of your dog. We all know what we don't want our dogs to do, but it is much more helpful to actually consider what we do want them to do. Dogs pick up on our thoughts and feelings very easily, so if you are giving him a positive instruction from the subconscious level, it will help him understand what is expected. This pattern of thinking also means rephrasing what you say to yourself and to others when you are talking about your dog. Don't say 'I'm training Joey not to jump up', or 'I'm training him not to run away.' Instead say, 'I'm training Joey to stay quiet when people arrive', and 'I'm training Joey to come back to me when I call him'. Remember that thoughts, and the words that express them, are as important as your actions, and all of them can be used to achieve the good behaviour that you are aiming for. Young dogs are more compliant to being

MAKING THE NEGATIVE POSITIVE

Visualize and think about the positive outcomes for each negative situation:

Negative = Barking at the doorbell.
Positive = Sitting quietly in his basket when the door bell sounds.

Negative = Barking when you go out.
Positive = Lying in his basket when you shut the front door.

Negative = Jumping up.
Positive = Greeting people by coming up to them and sniffing their knees.

Negative = Pulling on the lead.
Positive = Walking at your side.

Negative = Not coming back when called.
Positive = Running back towards you as you call his name.

trained and learning new behaviour, but it is not impossible to train older dogs; it may just take longer.

Know what you want

Before any dog can be obedient to you, you need to decide what it is you want them to do, and how you would like them to do it. You need to be clear about the behaviour or response that you want from them from the start. If you are wishy-washy or uncertain, for instance knowing that you don't want him on the sofa, but not really caring where else he is, it is going to be more difficult for both of you. It will be much more effective to communicate 'I want you to be in your basket', which is a clear and definite

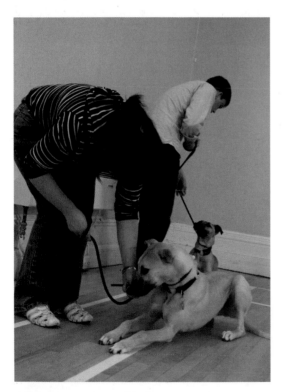

Always reward good behaviour when you are training your dog.

command. This will give your dog a much clearer understanding of where he should be, and a better chance of learning the ropes. Giving him boundaries and rules doesn't mean that you are being strict and harsh; it actually gives your dog more freedom to relax. It means that he won't feel anxious about what he should or shouldn't be doing. This is where teaching your dog good manners comes in. For example, you need to train your dog not to push through doors before you, or jump out of the car before you tell him to. These rules are not just for good manners, they are also to stop him running out onto the road and potentially causing an accident. Another example is jumping up at people and possibly scaring them. This training has nothing to do with not allowing your dog to be 'dominant' over you, it is just good manners and for safety reasons; common sense really.

Calmness and consistency

These are the key to a contented and well-behaved dog. As well as being consistent in your own behaviour to him, it is vital that all members of the family, and everyone who interacts with your dog, follow the same rules. It's no good if some members of the family allow him on the sofa, and others don't, or if sometimes he is allowed upstairs, but not always.

The next thing to clear up from the start is that your dog won't have an innate understanding of right and wrong in the same way that we understand these terms. So he won't know that it is 'bad manners' to jump up, or bound onto the sofa, unless he has been taught that this is frowned upon. As they are not human and don't have the same social rules as we do, dogs obviously don't know that 'stealing', 'destroying' and getting things mucky are innately 'wrong'. Therefore it is down to training that he will learn what is acceptable behaviour and what is not, in all circumstances. This is where consistency comes in again; if he is not allowed on chairs, this rule should apply to all chairs, whether he is at home or elsewhere. Training is the same too. Practise sit and recall in all sorts of different places so that your dog associates sitting with you saying it and the reward, rather than just doing it when he hears you say it in one particular spot. Being calm, patient and consistent is the key to training him. This way you will be demonstrating to him that you are a good role model. If you act erratically and inconsistently, your dog will be confused and not inclined to follow or obey, because he is anxious and unsettled about what could happen next.

Positive reinforcement

How can we turn negative behaviour patterns into positive ones? This is done through a training method called 'positive reinforcement', whereby the desired behaviour is rewarded. Obviously this is often harder to put into practice than it sounds, because some issues can be pretty complex. In these instances, and especially if there are potentially dangerous behaviours, including biting, expert help must be sought as soon as possible.

Dogs generally see things as being exciting or boring, safe or dangerous, rather than right or wrong, good or bad. They do not plan or think ahead, they base their actions on what usually happens straight after they have acted. Looking at situations like this from the dog's perspective, we can start to understand how their behaviours are shaped and what we can do to un-shape them. Positive reinforcement means rewarding your dog for a good or desired behaviour with something that they highly value, usually food, but also attention or a toy. In other words, giving your dog something he values in exchange for him doing something you value. Because dogs are so clever and make connections so readily, the timing of the reward is of crucial importance; otherwise they will link the wrong behaviour with the treat. Your dog will only be able to associate the reward with the action if it is given at exactly the same time. For example, if your dog takes ages coming back when you call him, and when he eventually does you pull and jerk him on the lead and tell him off for ignoring you, he will associate your negative response with his coming back. This will mean that next time you call him, he won't be tempted to come back because he associates this with a negative experience. It is the same with house-training; you have to be ready with the reward as soon as your puppy performs in the garden, so that he links peeing outside with a treat. Also remember that you need to practise your dog's training in a lot of different environments but keep your voice, the words you use and the rewards consistent. On this note, be aware that many dog treats are full of colours, preservatives and mood-changing E numbers, all best avoided if you want optimum concentration and behaviour from your dog. You can use some of your dog's dry kibble food as the reward, taken from his daily rations so as not to cause weight gain, or you could offer him a piece of carrot or a chunk of apple. Try and vary the rewards you use to keep your dog's interest and attention. This is another reason for keeping some of his toys out of everyday circulation, as in this way they will have a higher value as a reward.

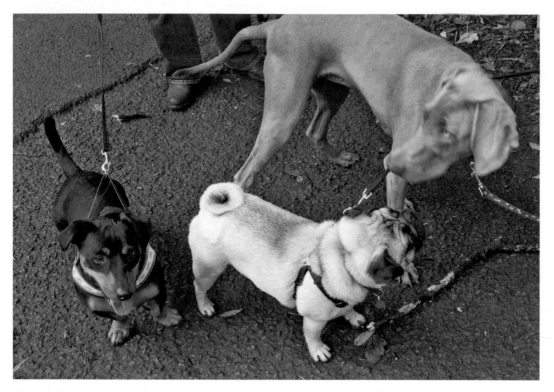

Keep training sessions short and sweet.

Rest and recuperation

Another thing to bear in mind is not to overdo the training of young puppies. Remember that they have so many new experiences and routines to get used to that they also need plenty of time to rest and recover, both mentally and physically. Related to this, make sure that training sessions are done when your dog is calm. Don't try and train him when he is wired up by playing or if he is overexcited. Stop a training session if he has had enough. Stressed or tired dogs cannot process new learning experiences and it will not be an effective way to teach him. Make sure that there are as few distractions as possible when you are training him. Gradually build these in, until he will respond in a normal situation where there are usually lots of other things going on. For example, begin your dog's training in a quiet place at home, where there are just the two of you. Then, when he has mastered what it is you are teaching him to do here, start to ask him to do it in places where there are increasingly more distractions, such as the garden and then the park. It's better to do several shorter training sessions a day than one long one.

Keep calm and carry on

How about stopping an unwanted behaviour? Fundamentally, this consists of ignoring it and rewarding your dog when he does the opposite, or desired, behaviour. You will also need to work on removing as many of the triggers for the unwanted behaviour as possible. But if the trigger is an unavoidable, everyday thing such as the postman or the doorbell, you will need to try your best to stop your dog being exposed to it, for as long as you can, before gradually reintroducing it in a very controlled manner. Your dog needs to learn that these triggers, such as the doorbell and the postman, are nothing to worry about. It is also very important to remember that most dogs crave attention and value it very highly, so they interpret a 'telling off', even a 'no', as a positive interaction. This is why ignoring is a very useful tool. Ways of ignoring bad behaviour might include just carrying on with what you are doing, or even leaving the room.

Some key concepts to be clear about are when to stroke and pat your dog, in other words reassure him, and when to ignore him. Stroking, patting and talking to him are of course all positive interactions and indicate that whatever the dog is doing at that exact time is good and what you want him to do. This is why you are discouraged from patting and stroking to 'reassure' your dog when he is anxious, as he will interpret this as a 'well done' for acting in an anxious way. An example of this is around fireworks night, when a lot of dogs feel frightened and are shaking and want to get on your lap. However, by stroking an anxious dog and allowing him up on your lap for a cuddle you are giving him a sign of reassurance, which he will take to mean that he was right to be scared of the fireworks. Instead, this is a time for ignoring an anxious dog, or just carrying on as if everything is fine, as indeed fireworks are. This is mirroring the behaviour of your dog's mother, who wouldn't run away or fuss over her pups

when they were frightened of something that was not a threat; instead she would just carry on as if nothing untoward was happening.

Training aids

There are various aids to help with training your dog. These range from the excellent to the truly awful. Clicker training is on the excellent side. This is a little gadget that you can hold in your hand that makes a click sound; you use it as soon as your dog does something you want him to do. Initially you will need to both click and reward your dog. After a while you will find that the click alone will be enough, as your dog will associate the click with having been rewarded. The shock and citronella squirting collars are at the other end of the spectrum. They are negative training tools that make the dog associate a particular behaviour with a feeling of pain. They just act to reinforce fear and anxiety in the dog, and are paving the way to further, often worse, behaviour problems. Hence there is no justification for using these aids under any circumstance and no expert would suggest using them. To combat unwanted behaviour in your dog, it is vital to understand why he is doing it. From there, it is necessary to work out how to change the situation and if possible remove its triggers or causes. By doing this you are addressing the root cause of the problem rather than just suppressing the resulting behaviour.

Qualified dog trainers and behaviourists

At the time of writing, the accreditation for dog trainers and behaviourists is undergoing major upheaval. Therefore the best advice at present is to seek the advice of your vet, and ask them for a referral or a recommendation.

4 THE PUPPY

Getting a new puppy is very exciting and a lot of fun, but at the same time it's a big responsibility and will require a lot of time and patience. After all, your new puppy is a blank canvas and it's going to be your job to make sure that he turns into a friendly, well-behaved adult. His future mental, emotional and physical health will be largely dependent on how you treat and care for him as a puppy. This chapter will guide you through the most important steps in puppy care, including how to cope on the first night you get him home. It will also cover other key aspects, such as socialization and feeding, as well as training and play. Finally, there is a section on common puppy ailments and suggested complementary treatments.

THE EARLY DAYS

At the breeder's

It is not an exaggeration to say that the first few weeks of your puppy's life are fundamental in forming his adult temperament. That's why choosing where you get your puppy from is very important. His experiences at the breeder's during the first few weeks, while he is just starting to develop and learn, will mould your puppy's responses and behaviour patterns for later life. This is because his 'socialization period' starts from around three weeks of age, when his eyes open. This period is the important stage between around three and sixteen weeks when your puppy is learning to recognize and interact with the world around him. In fact this recognition starts even before your pup's eyes open. Studies where half of a litter were exposed to the scent of humans in the first few days of their lives found that later on these pups were much more

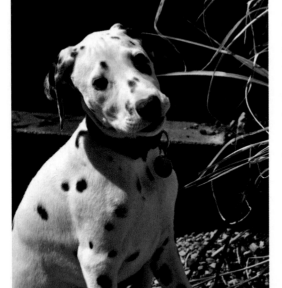

Getting a new puppy is a lot of fun.

engaged with human interaction than those without the very early contact. Because this familiarization and socialization starts so early, his life at the breeder's plays a key role in your puppy's emotional development. It is down to them to make sure that the puppies are exposed to everyday comings and goings, and the sights, sounds and smells of family life. The most important factor when choosing a puppy is to match what his home at the breeder's was like with his future lifestyle with you. So if you have young children and a hectic home life, then make sure that you find a breeder whose puppies have been brought up in a busy family situation, similar to your own. However, it works the other way too. For instance if your dog will have a relatively quiet life with you, then it pays to get a puppy from an environment where there has been less stimulation and activity. In fact, nurturing, or lack of it, in the puppy's early life is one of the most crucial factors that help to form his temperament and character as an adult. This goes along with current thinking in human psychology which suggests that it is most certainly nurture rather than nature which makes us into the adults we become.

Your puppy

Choosing your own puppy from the litter is of course a matter of per-sonal choice. However, it makes sense to choose one that looks lively, is interacting and interested in what is going on, is of a good average size and has a shiny, clean coat. All of these are signs that the puppy has sufficient 'qi' (as explained below in 'In the genes'), and consequently the potential for good long-term health. Spending time with the litter will help you to bond with, and choose, a particular puppy. One

more thing you may want to bear in mind in the planning stages of getting a puppy is that in the wild they would usually be born in the spring. This ensured that they could profit from the warmer weather, growing up and playing outside the den, and is why spring-born puppies were usually healthier. Therefore, if your circumstances permit it, consider all the benefits of getting your pup in the spring. If nothing else, it will make all those necessary house-training trips to the garden in the small hours a lot more pleasant if the weather is warmer. Finally, be aware of the pitfalls of taking time off work when you get your new puppy, as he will then need to adapt to a new routine once you go back to work. This is often when problems such as separation anxiety can begin.

Bringing him home: the first night

Your first forty-eight hours with your new puppy sets up his relationship with you, and his reactions to the world in general, for life. Therefore starting off on the right foot is of prime importance. Remember he is only a baby and be calm, patient and consistent in how you treat him. Preparation for your puppy's first night in his new home is important. He will have been used to sleeping with his mum and siblings in a warm nest, so try and simulate this by giving him a snug bed with familiar blankets that smell of his family. Provide some background sound, such as a ticking clock or a radio, as total silence will feel quite strange after sleeping with half a dozen other puppies. Where your puppy sleeps that first night is crucial; it needs to be the same place that you want him to sleep as an adult. If this is in your bedroom, that's fine as long as you always want him to sleep in your bedroom. It's equally impor-

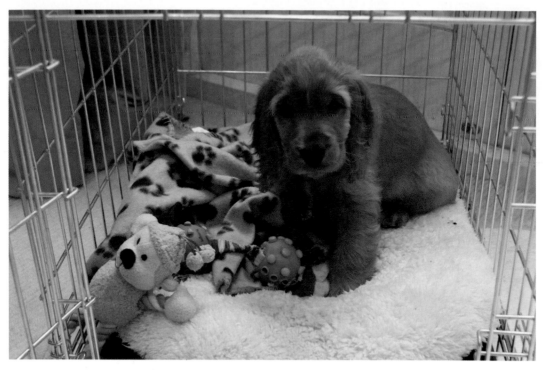

Where your puppy sleeps on his first night is crucial.

tant not to pet or console your puppy if he cries, however tempted you are, as this is one of the reasons that people end up with dogs that howl and cry all night. Of course, you will need to take him out for a pee during the night, but try and coordinate this with a time he is not crying. When you do take him out to the toilet, try not to fuss or stroke your puppy, as this will distract him from doing his business. Until he is house-trained, you may need to set your alarm clock so that you can wake up regularly to take your puppy outside to the toilet during the night. Although some of these instructions may sound mean and strict, puppies thrive on routine and consistency and will settle into their new home much more quickly and contentedly this way.

Socialization

'Socialization' is a term that means 'getting your puppy used to things'. This will have begun when he was still at the breeder's and should continue as soon as your puppy arrives at his new home with you. The most crucial time to get him used to new things is up until your puppy is about sixteen weeks old, but exposure after this point shouldn't stop. He needs to learn that all the different sights, smells and sounds that go on in the world around him are nothing to be worried about. It's a good idea to have a pocketful of treats when you are introducing your puppy to new people, such as people with big hats, or pushing bikes, so that they can then offer him a treat when they say 'hello'. Enlisting the help of a

CHECKLIST FOR THE FIRST NIGHT WITH YOUR NEW PUPPY

- Leave your puppy with his mum and family for as long as feasible, if he is being well socialized and it is a good match for his new home with you.
- Make sure he has a familiar blanket or toy.
- A hot water bottle, wrapped in towel or blanket for warmth.
- The sound of ticking clock or a radio on low.
- Start him sleeping in the same place he will sleep as an adult.
- Don't console him if he wakes and cries.
- Rescue Remedy in his water or food if he is upset.
- Aconite, the homeopathic remedy for shock.

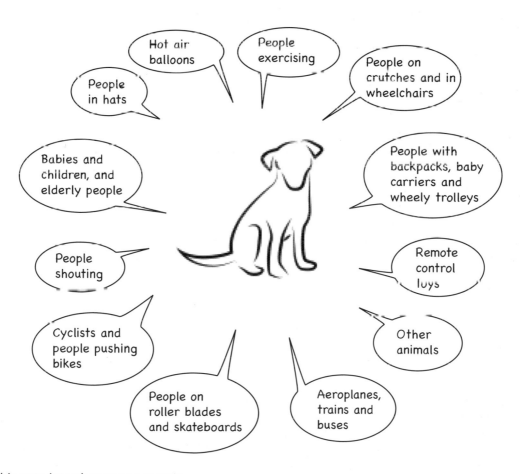

Things to introduce your puppy to.

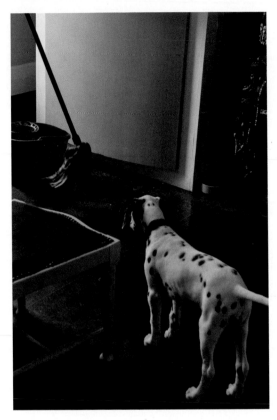

Get your puppy used to a wide range of everyday things, such as mopping.

calm, confident, well-socialized older dog to go with you is also an excellent idea. This will help your puppy pick up good calm vibes from him and thus boost his confidence. It's important to realize that if your puppy starts to show any signs of anxiety, such as trembling, cowering, or licking his lips, or seems in any way overwhelmed by his new experiences, you should not force him nearer but just head for home. Equally, although it seems natural to do so, don't pet or reassure your puppy in these situations, as you would be inadvertently reinforcing his

fearful response. Just be bright and breezy and take him swiftly past the thing he is anxious about.

FEEDING

Food is the raw material, the building block, for every cell in the body. This is why your puppy's diet is of fundamental importance to his growth and development into a strong and healthy adult. Along with his exercise, diet will have the greatest effect on your puppy's bones and joints, and hence his size, shape, strength and fitness as an adult. With the consequences of early nutrition having such important knock-on effects into adulthood, choosing the right diet for your puppy is essential. Puppies grow quickly in the first few months, so puppyhood is the most nutritionally demanding time in his life. The diet of large-breed puppies (those with an adult weight of over 20 kg) in particular must be perfectly balanced to allow for smooth and consistent growth until maturity. Although exact requirements cannot be given, as each puppy will differ depending on his breed, exercise routine and metabolic rate, as a general rule their nutritional needs can be divided into two main phases: the fast growth rate of the young puppy, followed at about five months of age by the slightly slower rate of the adolescent. Being aware that growth is a two-stage process is of particular importance in large and giant breeds of dog. They will need particular attention to their diet during adolescence, to ensure that it is tailored to this slower but more sustained growth phase. Weighing your puppy regularly, every few weeks, will help you to make sure that he is growing steadily and not becoming overweight.

Different requirements

Whatever their breed, because they are growing rapidly puppies have a higher requirement for protein, energy and calcium than an adult. In fact from birth until he reaches half his adult weight, your puppy will have around double the daily energy requirements of an adult. For the rest of his growth, until he reaches his mature size at around twelve months old, he will need about 50 per cent more than the adult. This is why puppy foods were developed, to take account of these varying needs and cater for them. If you are home cooking, you will still need to take these different energy and protein needs into account and prepare meals accordingly. Although there is this increased requirement for calories and protein, overfeeding during his growing phase is one of the most common pitfalls of puppy feeding. Obesity will predispose your puppy to skeletal problems, especially in large-breed dogs. Calcium is a key component of the bones of the skeleton, hence your puppy's higher requirement as he is growing. However, it is crucial that this is provided in exactly the correct proportion to the other key bone mineral, phosphorus. This will be provided in proprietary diets, so there will be no need to worry. Again, however, if you are feeding your puppy on a home-prepared diet make sure that the recipe that you are following has known ratios of these elements, and that the diet has been well tried and tested for your particular breed of puppy.

Mealtimes

In addition to what you are feeding him, the other important difference between feeding a puppy compared to an adult dog is the number of meals he needs

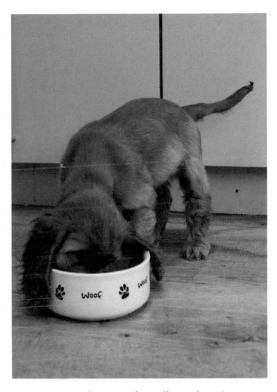

A puppy needs several small meals a day.

every day. Puppies have small stomachs and a digestive tract that is just getting used to solid foods, so they need to be fed little and often. The breeder will usually provide you with a small supply of the food that they have weaned your puppy onto. This is useful because it will be one less new thing for him to adjust to in his new home, and hence one less trigger for an upset tummy. So he can be kept on his usual food for the first few days, and if you are going to change him onto something else, this can be done gradually thereafter. Gradual transitions are always recommended because it will take a few days for the natural bacteria in your puppy's intestinal tract to adjust

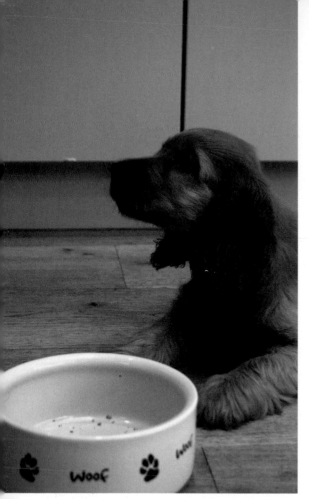

Use ceramic bowls for food and water.

bowl is ideal; as always, plastic is to be avoided.

As for the practicalities of feeding your puppy, it is good practice to remove any uneaten food after each meal. This saves grazing and a picky appetite and also stops the food going off and spoiling. Your puppy will then learn that he needs to eat at mealtimes. It's a good idea to get him used to having his bowl touched, or even moved, when he is eating, to stop him becoming possessive over it. The best way of doing this is just to add a little extra food to it while he is eating. If you have more than one dog then do feed them from separate bowls, and some-times even in separate rooms, as compet-itiveness during eating can result in digestive upsets. Don't worry if your puppy picks up some of his food and takes it away from his bowl to eat it; it is natural in the wild for wolf cubs to tear off a chunk of meat from the kill and go off and eat it on their own, away from the pack.

No milk please

Puppies, just like adult dogs, need to have constant access to fresh water. Some people advocate filtered water but this is not essential. The bottom line is that whatever is good enough for the people in the household to be drinking is good enough for the dog. Contrary to what some breeders still suggest, once they are weaned puppies no longer have the capacity to be able to digest milk. This is why, although he may like it, giving your puppy milk is not good for him and will be likely to cause an upset tummy.

and adapt to his changing food supply. This is partly the reason why puppies are so often affected by diarrhoea when they first arrive at their new home; there are just so many adjustments to make: new family, new environment, and new food. Using probiotic supplements that are full of the 'good bugs' he needs can help to alleviate intestinal upsets at this stage. Puppies are usually fed about four times a day until they reach three months of age, when it can be reduced down to three, and then twice daily at about six months. Using a ceramic or stainless steel

PLAYTIME AND EXERCISE

Playtime is crucial to puppies because it teaches them how to interact with you, as well as with other dogs. Different types of play are important as natural outlets for your puppy's in-built need to chase, capture and chew. In the wild this would of course have been sheep, rabbits and deer, but hopefully for most pet dogs, balls and plastic toys have taken their place! Don't forget that playtime isn't just 'down-time'; your puppy actually needs the mental and physical satisfaction of performing these activities as part of his balanced development.

The Taoist tradition, which is part of Traditional Chinese Medicine, one of the most complete preventive health care systems in the world, has a saying that 'Flowing water never stagnates, active hinges never rust'. This explains why exercise is recognized as vital in maintaining an optimal balance in both the mental and physical aspects of every dog's health. On the physical side, regular exercise will keep your puppy's joints flexible and his muscles and ligaments strong, thus helping to prevent injury. There is a popular belief that puppies and young dogs, especially large breeds, should not be 'over-exercised', with some people suggesting no off-lead exercise at all for young dogs. Now, while it is of course sensible for puppies not to overdo it on walks with too much running around, preventing any exercise at all would be extreme. You should simply trust your common sense with regard to how much exercise your puppy needs, depending on his level of fitness and what he is used to. Don't forget that as a youngster this is the most important time of life for him to be able to enjoy running about, playing and chasing. This is all part of 'puppy school', and by doing moderate, sensible and regular exercise, he will stay fit and strong. In fact, a more important risk factor for large-breed puppies is over-exercising rather than over-feeding. Obesity puts increased strain on his joints, so pay attention to overfeeding as well as over-exercising. The renowned herbalist and dog breeder Juliette de Bairacli Levi was a huge fan of rearing puppies with plentiful access to the outdoors, explaining how sunlight provides vitamins A and D that are essential for growth. She also said that being able to lick fresh dew from the grass in the mornings was a natural, healthy tonic for dogs that they will seek out themselves by instinct.

Chewing and teething

Puppies enjoy playing a range of different games: using tug or chew toys, looking for hidden treats, as well as the ever-popular game of fetching a ball. Each type of pastime or different toy helps your puppy to learn a different skill, and can be especially useful at different stages of his development. For example, chewing toys can be used around the time of teething to ease any pain and discomfort in his mouth. Your puppy should have a full set of temporary baby teeth by the time he is eight weeks old. He will then shed these as his adult teeth come through at between three to six months of age. Also, by offering him chew toys you will be making it less likely that your puppy will choose his own items to chew, such as your shoes. TTouch (see Chapter 1) can be a useful tool to help ease any pain and discomfort associated with teething, and can also be helpful in getting him used to the toothbrush. You will need to start getting your puppy used to having his teeth brushed as early as possible, because he will need them brushed every day if he is going to be fed anything other than a bones and raw meat diet. TTouch is where small circles

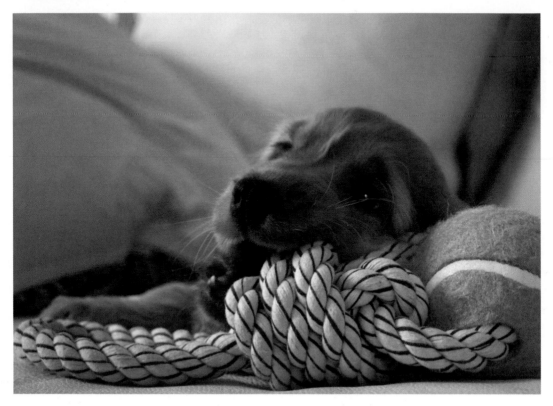

Puppies love chew toys.

are made with your fingertips around your puppy's mouth and on his lips, to massage and relax his mouth and jaw. However, chew toys are not just for puppies, they are beneficial for adult dogs too as the mechanical action of chewing, along with the saliva itself, helps to reduce plaque buildup on the teeth. Begin to brush your puppy's teeth regularly as early as possible. First use just your finger and some toothpaste, then a finger brush, and finally, when your puppy is comfortable having these in his mouth, use a soft toothbrush. Regular brushing removes plaque and helps to ensure healthy teeth and gums (*see*

Chapter 9). The addition of a sprinkling of finely chopped parsley or a pinch of seaweed to his food will also help reduce plaque and keep your dog's breath smelling sweeter.

Throwing balls and sticks

There is always much debate as to whether it is advisable to throw sticks for your dog, or indeed to allow him to chew them. Although it seems the most natural thing in the world to chuck a stick for him, the problems that arise if your dog catches it awkwardly and it lodges in his mouth or throat can be serious. Vets do not support the practice of throwing sticks for dogs because they all too often see the consequences of these antics, which can include life-threatening injuries. Of course it isn't just sticks that can get lodged in the throat; if caught awkwardly, balls can get stuck too. Avoiding sticks, and otherwise being careful in what you choose to throw for your dog when playing these games, can at least minimize the risks.

Play biting

Make sure you balance your puppy's play-times with calm activities and rest. Above all, if play gets too vigorous or play biting too painful (puppies' baby teeth are like needles), then it's time to stop. They will then learn that using their teeth quickly puts an end to the game, which should be incentive enough to stop. This is also what they will learn when they play with other puppies and older dogs, usually getting a sharp telling-off if they bite too hard.

ADOLESCENCE

Adolescent dogs, just like teenage kids, can be a handful. When young dogs reach around six months old their hormones start to kick in and the obedience and manners that you have spent the last six months teaching them can sometimes go out of the window. This is

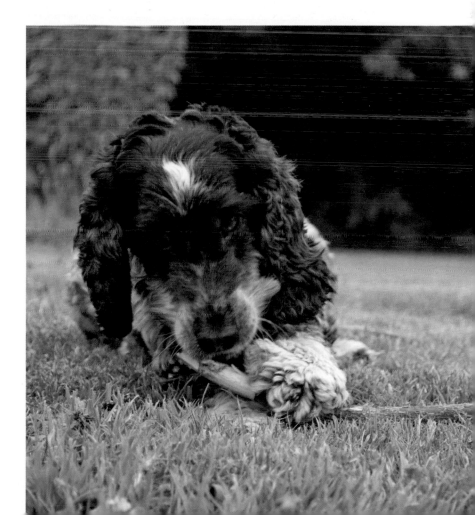

Chewing and catching sticks can be dangerous.

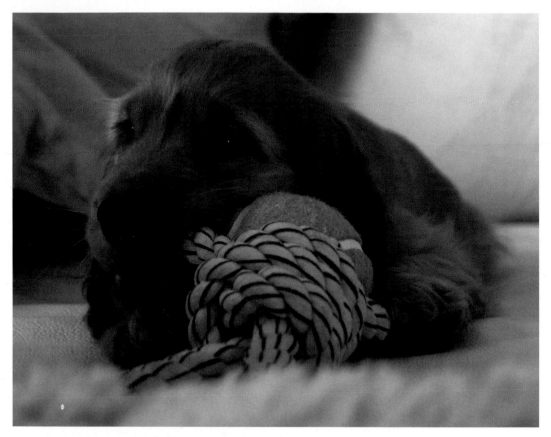

Puppies' baby teeth are as sharp as needles.

normal. Dogs don't really reach emotional and mental maturity until they are eighteen months to two years old, later than they reach physical maturity. So don't despair if you think that your youngster will never learn to sit quietly, or has frequent lapses in attention; this is to be expected until they are a grown up. Patience and consistency in your expectations are the key throughout puppyhood. But don't forget that problems are not always entirely down to your dog's surge in hormones; make sure that you are consistent with your training and attentiveness too.

Bitches and seasons

Bitches' hormones begin to circulate from around six months, so this is when gender differences between male and female youngsters start to become more obvious. Her first season can be any time from six months. This is usually mild and can go completely unremarked, or you may notice swelling of her vulva and dripping blood. Unless you want her mated (not recommended at her first season), keep your bitch under a very watchful eye and any interested males at bay. She may become clingy while she is in season, wanting more fuss and cuddles, and may also begin to 'mother' a toy or a sock or cushion, which she will carry around in her mouth as if it were a puppy. She may become quite protective of it, and may also try and make a nest in her bed. These are all natural instincts, and just leaving her to it is the best advice. However, in some cases this can go one step further and the bitch gets what is called a 'false pregnancy' where her mammary glands develop and she may even produce a little milk. This is a left-over trait from the time of her wolf ancestor, when several females in the pack would come into season at the same time as the breeding female had puppies. They would then share the suckling of this litter between them. A false pregnancy is usually mild and clears up on its own after a few days. However, if it doesn't, have her checked by the vet to make sure that this is the correct diagnosis. There are several effective homeopathic remedies to treat false pregnancy, most commonly one called Pulsatilla. A homeopathic vet would be able to prescribe this, or a more suitable remedy, in such situations.

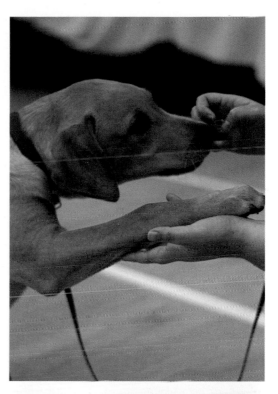

Males usually begin to cock their legs to pee at around six months too, and may start to become more boisterous or competitive with other males of the same size. It is at around this time, at six months of age, that neutering of males and females is usually carried out.

The Bach Flower Remedy Walnut helps with times of change, such as during adolescence. Add two drops to your dog's water bowl, changed daily, for three weeks.

TOP: *Train your puppy using rewards.*

BOTTOM: *Patience and consistency are crucial throughout puppyhood.*

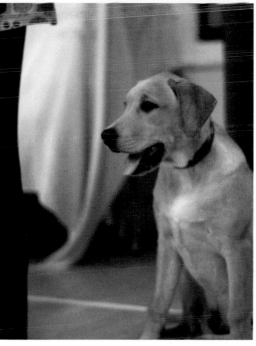

INHERITED CONDITIONS

In the genes

According to Traditional Chinese Medicine philosophy, an individual's lifelong health is down to a special form of energy in their body called 'jing' or 'essence'. They have a finite amount of this energy, which is gradually used up throughout life. The amount and quality of this inherited vitality is a reflection of the energy, both emotional and physical, of the parents at the time of conception. Jing, according to TCM, is the underlying factor predisposing us to health. Thus a puppy with enough jing will have a long life free of any untoward health problems, whereas a puppy whose parents were weak, old or ill will have poor 'jing' energy and will be the runt of the litter, a 'poor-doer' and prone to illness. Jing is similar to the Western idea of genes and genetic make-up. Jing cannot be topped up or added to later in life, it is finite; this is why making sure you choose a healthy puppy from the start is so important. You can make sure that your puppy has plenty of jing by assessing both him and his parents. Check that he is active and energetic, that his tongue is moist and pink, his coat is shiny, his eyes bright and that he doesn't have diarrhoea or any other health problem. As regards the parents, check that they are bright and healthy and of sound temperament and have been well treated. It is also important that they are not too old, nor have had many litters, as jing is lost throughout life, so that older dogs necessarily have less jing to pass on to their pups. For the same reasons, puppies from larger litters may potentially have less jing, but only if the bitch is older or in weaker health. Young, fit bitches should be able to have a good number of strong, healthy pups.

Do try and meet the parents when you are choosing your puppy so that you get an idea of their character and temperament, as well as their state of health. Homeopathic philosophy also places great value on the health of the parents when it comes to the future health and fitness of their puppies. Here the genetic susceptibilities are called miasms. This is the term that homeopaths use to describe the main patterns of symptoms that they see in people, and animals, when they are ill. It helps them to use the correct homeopathic remedy for their patient, based on the principles of 'like cures like' (*see* Chapter 1).

Of course, in Western medicine we can relate the ideas behind jing and miasms to what we know about genes and inherited disorders. We realize that some conditions are passed along in families through the genes. It is clear that pedigree dogs are more likely to suffer from such genetic disorders simply because they come from a smaller gene pool. Each particular breed has a susceptibility to certain inherited diseases or conditions, and these should be looked into while you are considering which dog to get. Information is available on various websites and through the Kennel Club, as well as from your local vet. Conscientious and reputable breeders will be well aware of the potential problems in their chosen breed and will carry out the necessary screening tests for these, such as hip scoring for many large breeds and eye tests for breeds such as collies and spaniels. Don't forget that it's not only physical conditions that are inherited; temperament too can be genetic. Families of dogs with known behaviour problems should not be bred from.

Your vet will examine your new puppy carefully on his first visit, as some inher-

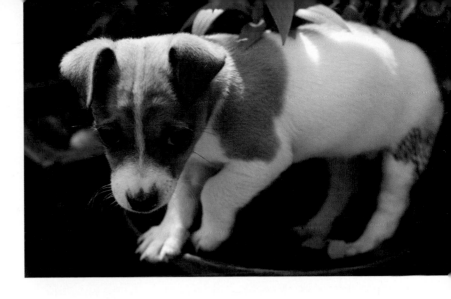

This little puppy has plenty of jing.

ited conditions can be picked up at an early stage. This is part of the routine check over from nose to tail, listening to his heart, looking in his eyes, and feeling him all over, so that any problems are picked up as soon as possible.

MICROCHIPPING

It may be around this time of first vaccinations and first veterinary check up that you get your puppy microchipped. A microchip is an electronic chip about the size of a grain of rice that is inserted, by injection, just under the skin between the shoulder blades. It consists of a unique number that links to a computer database that contains all your contact details and basic information about your dog. Therefore if he gets lost and ends up at a vet's or rescue centre, by scanning the chip they will find your contact details and you will stand the best chance of being reunited. Microchips are also a mandatory part of the process for taking your dog abroad under the pet passport scheme. The main concerns around microchipping relate to the permanent insertion of a foreign body into an animal's system and any potential problems in the chip itself. However, in the last ten years or so, when microchipping has become commonplace, there have been very few problems with the thousands of microchips placed in dogs every day. Weighing up both the actual and theoretical health risks against the possibility of your dog being lost, or even stolen, the benefits of microchipping far outweigh the risks.

PUPPY HEALTH AND COMMON AILMENTS

For several reasons puppies can be more susceptible to illnesses than adults. They are under more stress due to leaving their mum and siblings; then there is the change in digestive processes associated with weaning, and often a change of diet. They are also getting used to a new home, new people and have many new things to learn. All of these events are putting extra strain on the puppy's immune system, making him more susceptible to illness. However, in homeopathic terms, the vital force (or the innate strength of the immune and rebalancing system) is strong in puppies. This means that given the right help and supportive care, they should naturally be able to bounce back from most illnesses more quickly. You too are going through a steep learning curve, especially if it is your first dog, and you are a 'new parent'. This means that you may well be unsure about whether any sign or symptom that your puppy develops is serious or not. Enlisting the help of friends and family that have had dogs before is useful, as is checking and chatting through any worrying symptoms with your vet. The list below is a mini guide to some of the most common ailments in puppies, alongside tips for safe home treatment. (A more comprehensive list of conditions that affect adults, as well as puppies, can be found in Chapter 9.)

Always remember that you can't be too careful when it comes to your new puppy's health. So if in doubt about any symptom, it's much better to have the vet check him over and reassure you that it's nothing to worry about, than have a sleepless night not knowing.

Diarrhoea

This is by far the most common problem in puppies brought to the vet's. It is commonly due to the fact that their digestive system is having to adapt to solid food as well as get used to a new diet. Worms or a bacterial infection can also cause diarrhoea in puppies, or it could be due to eating something he shouldn't, perhaps out of the dustbin.

If, as is commonly the case with diarrhoea, your puppy remains bright and bouncy and has a good appetite, then do the following.

In mild cases

Bland food, little and often. In adult dogs the first step is usually to starve them for twenty-four hours with just water, or honey-water available, allowing the digestive system the chance to rest and repair. However, as puppies have a higher metabolism, such a long period of fasting is not recommended, and they should usually continue to be fed throughout the diarrhoea. Offer small meals little and often, about a tablespoon of food six to eight times a day. Bland food, such as chicken and rice (or millet) is the order of the day. Continue this diet for a few days and then gradually reintroduce his usual food if all is going well.

Electrolyte fluid You can also offer your puppy an oral rehydration solution to drink, preferably from your vet's. This will help to prevent him suffering any mineral or electrolyte imbalances due to the diarrhoea. This will also help the gastrointestinal tract to repair itself, and so speed recovery.

Probiotics Another way of supporting your puppy's system and helping to resolve the diarrhoea is the use of pre- and probiotics. These will repopulate his digestive system with the 'good bugs' that he needs in order to digest his food properly, and which may well be depleted or out of sync if he has had diarrhoea. Some people give their puppies a probiotic supplement (such as lactobacilli) for a few weeks as a matter of course, to help prevent diarrhoea and other gastrointestinal upsets, when they arrive at their new home. Vets often prescribe proprietary pastes or powders that contain both probiotics and kaolin. This helps to re-establish the intestinal bugs, and the kaolin is a clay-like mineral that helps make formed stools again.

At the vet's
Taking your puppy to the vets is important if the diarrhoea has blood in it, if he is off his food, if he has a painful or

bloated tummy, or if he is vomiting or seems depressed and lethargic. Your vet will be able to check him all over and make sure that he doesn't have a temperature, isn't dehydrated and doesn't have any sign of a blockage or other problem in his tummy. If he has none of these things, your vet will be able to assure you that home treatment and TLC is fine, and to give you rehydration and probiotic supplements as necessary. On the other hand, if your vet has concerns he may admit your puppy for treatment. Taking in a sample of your puppy's diarrhoea, in a plastic bag or jar, will often be helpful for the vet, who will then be able to send it to the lab for analysis. They will check whether the diarrhoea is due to bacteria or a parasite (an intestinal worm, such as roundworm), or other common puppy diarrhoea bugs (such as cocciddia or Giardia). It is important to get this diagnostic test done if the diarrhoea is in any way ongoing, because it may require specific veterinary medications, such as wormers or antibiotics, to clear it up. This is also important because some of these diseases are zoontic, which means they can be passed on to people.

Conjunctivitis

This is the inflammation of the mucus membranes that surround the eye. If your puppy's eyes seem red or inflamed or if he has discharge from the inner corners of his eyes, then he may be suffering from conjunctivitis. He may also hold his eye or eyes shut, as if squinting or blinking, or rub at his face in discomfort. Conjunctivitis can be quite common in puppies, especially in breeds with a lot of skin folds on their faces or those with prominent eyes. A visit to the vet's is always needed with any eye problem, however minor it may seem. This is because eye conditions can potentially be very serious, and the sooner they are treated the better the prognosis. So it is not a case of trying to manage an eye complaint with home treatment first and then having it checked if it's not getting better. Have your puppy's eyes checked over as soon as you spot a problem. (*See* Chapter 9 for complementary treatments for conjunctivitis.)

Skin rash

It's not uncommon for puppies to develop rashes on the hairless parts of the body, such as the tummy, armpits, face or groin. These may come up suddenly, perhaps due to a contact allergy, something that your puppy has been lying on or brushed against in the environment, or even something you have washed him in. If it is more of an all-over symptom, then it is more likely to be a reaction to something that he has eaten, or a response to something that he has been exposed to that has caused a whole-body reaction, an allergic reaction. Some dietary ingredients, such as beef or wheat, have more potential for causing problems than others. So in some cases simply changing the diet is all that needs to be done. Often these rashes or patches of inflamed skin disappear as quickly as they come up, without any treatment. However, the use of topical aloe vera gel or lotion can be soothing and calming to the area and may help speed up recovery. Marigold, as a dried herb or as freshly picked flowers (crushed petals), added to the food is one of the best cleansing herbs, with antiseptic and healing properties. The homeopathic remedy Sulphur is commonly used for red and itchy skin, with one or two doses of a low potency (6c) usually enough. Of course, in any case where the rash or area of sore skin does not quickly resolve, or if it is painful or spreading, then your puppy needs to be taken for a veterinary check-up.

Ear problems

Puppies can sometimes suffer from sore and uncomfortable ears. Symptoms include shaking their heads, scratching at them, and resenting you touching their ears. The ear canals are lined with a very sensitive and delicate skin, easily traumatized by scratching. Irritated or inflamed ears tend to appear red and to have a blackish-brown crusty discharge. Ear problems can be part of a generalized skin condition (such as the rashes explained above), or may be due to ear mites (*Otodectes cyanotis*), or even something getting lodged in the ear canal, such as a grass seed. A trip to the vet's is undoubtedly necessary for any case of sore, irritated ears.

Ear mites

Ear mites live right down inside the ear canal, causing much itching and usually producing a lot of brown waxy debris. Your vet may be able to identify them by having a good look down your puppy's ear canal using a special instrument called an otoscope, and by taking a sample of the waxy discharge. Your puppy may need some conventional anti-parasitic medications to eradicate ear mites, as the herbal solution outlined in Chapter 9 may not be enough on its own. Any medicated drops should be used exactly according to the directions from the vet because mites go through life-cycles and adults need to be killed as they emerge over three weeks.

Being stepped on, tripped over or dropped

Unfortunately this happens – as puppies do tend to get into just the wrong place at the wrong time. Of course, in any such situation, take your puppy to the vet's to be thoroughly checked over to make sure that no internal damage has been done and that nothing is broken. The homeopathic remedy for shock, Aconite, should be given as soon as possible after the incident, just one dose of 30c. Arnica, the homeopathic remedy for trauma and bruising, can also be used in addition to the Aconite. The dose of Arnica will usually be 30c twice daily for a few days, depending on the extent of any injury. Your puppy may also need a few doses of Dr Bach's Rescue Remedy (for yourself too if you are shocked from stepping on your puppy), again to help him recover from the shock (see Chapter 1). None of these complementary remedies will affect the treatments that your vet may need to give your puppy, so they are suitable to give him in the car on the way to the vet's.

Reaction after first vaccination

Some puppies do appear to be affected by their vaccinations, especially the first one. They may seem a bit less energetic or off-colour for about twenty-four hours afterwards. If these symptoms go on for longer than this period, or are in any way more serious, then it's time for a check-up at the vet's to make sure he hasn't got a temperature or any other problem. The homeopathic remedy that is often given to animals that seem a little unwell after a vaccination, or indeed have any kind of reaction to it, is called Thuja. This can be given at a 30c potency up to twice a day, usually for two or three days after the vaccine. Some people use it routinely after a vaccination, whether there are any adverse effects in their animal or not.

5 PREVENTIVE HEALTH CARE

This chapter considers the role preventive health care plays in the overall, holistic treatment of your dog. Unfortunately, when it comes to preventive medicine, there is not a 'one size fits all' strategy that will suit every dog in every situation. That's why looking at the most likely health issues for your dog, alongside the range of possible treatment options, is important. By taking the holistic perspective on parasite control, for example, it will become clear that everyday common parasites such as fleas and worms should not cause a problem to a healthy dog. Comparing conventional treatments with the major complementary approaches to parasite control will help you find the most appropriate and effective way to manage fleas and worms in your dog.

This chapter also covers the process of taking your dog abroad, including details on the Pet Travel Scheme, and highlights a few of the health issues involved in foreign travel.

VACCINATION

Why is it important?
Vaccination is one of the most common veterinary procedures undertaken in dogs. There is no question that it plays an important role in preventing and controlling infectious diseases in the canine population. A vaccine works by stimulating the immune system so that it contains a blueprint of how to respond effectively should it be exposed to a given infection again in the future. So as not to actually

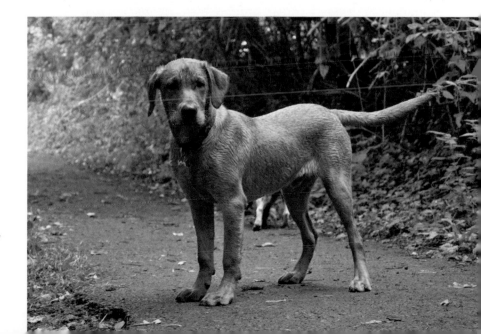

A healthy dog is not troubled by parasites.

cause disease in the dog, vaccines carry a modified or inactivated version of the infectious agent.

Which diseases do we vaccinate dogs against?

In the UK we routinely vaccinate all dogs against a handful of potentially lethal viruses that are present in the canine population. The most important of these are canine distemper, parvovirus and hepatitis, and these are given as your dog's core vaccine. Dogs also routinely receive vaccinations against the other diseases outlined below.

Distemper virus

One of the most serious canine diseases, potentially life-threatening, distemper attacks the respiratory, gastrointestinal and nervous systems. Thankfully, years of widespread vaccination have greatly reduced the prevalence of this disease. However, unvaccinated dogs, especially puppies, may still be at risk, therefore vaccination is important.

Parvovirus

Today this has replaced distemper as arguably the biggest threat among the infectious diseases to which your dog may be exposed. It is a life-threatening, highly infectious disease that causes severe vomiting, bloody diarrhoea and dehydration. The incidence of this infection varies, but it is still prevalent in many areas across the country, causing intermittent outbreaks of the disease. Because of its potentially deadly consequences, vaccination is crucial.

Infectious canine hepatitis

This virus most commonly affects puppies, but dogs of any age can be affected. There is some debate about how much of a risk this virus still causes; however, it is still a routine vaccination for most dogs.

Parainfluenza virus

This very contagious respiratory disease causes kennel cough. It is another routine vaccination for most dogs.

Leptospirosis

This is a bacterial disease that is mainly transmitted through the urine of infected wildlife. It is also a zoonotic disease, which means that it is transmissible to people. Infection can have potentially life-threatening consequences, so vaccination is important. However, to complicate matters, there are several subspecies of leptospirosis and there is some debate about whether the traditional vaccines protect dogs from the newer strains. Your vet should know which strains are most prevalent in your area and should therefore be using the most appropriate vaccine available.

We also vaccinate some, but not all, dogs against the following diseases, depending on the risk factors involved.

Kennel cough

This is a vaccine that contains protection against one of the major causes of this disease, Bordatella. It is an intra-nasal vaccine that is sprayed up your dog's nose. It may be a stipulation that your dog has a kennel cough vaccine in order to go to some boarding kennels.

Rabies

This is a viral disease affecting the central nervous system. It can affect all mammals, including humans, and is transmitted through a bite from an infected animal. Because this is not as yet endemic in this country, compulsory vaccination is not mandatory. This is only a requirement if you are taking your dog abroad, such as under the Pet Passport scheme.

When do we vaccinate puppies?

The usual protocol is for puppies to receive their vaccinations at between eight and twelve weeks of age. This is called a primary vaccination and it is given in two parts, with a few weeks between them. Each part will consist of just a single injection of a multi-agent vaccine. Your puppy will not have full protection for between one to two weeks after the second vaccine. While you still need to be vigilant about what you expose him to, you mustn't stop socializing your puppy during this period. Timing of the puppy vaccinations is important. If they are given too early, the immunity from the bitch may still be active in the puppy, which means that his vaccination will be less effective. If, on the other hand, they are left too late there may be a window of opportunity for infection. Your vet will usually follow a particular protocol that is matched to the level of disease risk in your area and is designed to offer your puppy maximum protection.

Note: The latest guidance from the World Small Animal Veterinary Association (WSAVA, 2010) advises that the primary vaccine should be given in three parts, with the final part at between fourteen and eighteen weeks of age. This is currently not routine in this country. Ask your vet about this, especially in view of parvovirus becoming endemic in some areas.

When do we vaccinate adult dogs?

After his puppy vaccines your dog will usually be revaccinated annually; this is called a booster. The booster will revaccinate your dog for the core diseases,

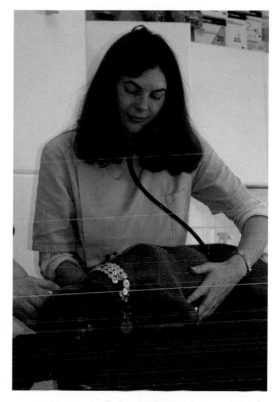

Regular veterinary health checks are important.

distemper, parvovirus and hepatitis, every three years, and the other components annually. Your vet will know from your dog's vaccination record which one he needs.

Are there any side effects to vaccination?

The main concerns related to vaccination are to do with over-vaccinating, in other words giving your dog too many boosters. There is a worry that repeated vaccination is linked to chronic disease. Revaccinating a dog that is already protected by a previous booster stimulates his immune system unnecessarily, does nothing to improve his resistance to the disease, and may increase the risk of adverse reaction. In addition, the common practice of giving multiple vaccines at the same time, as a single injection, has possible further negative consequences on your dog's finely tuned immune system. It is due to these concerns that most vaccine manufacturers reduced their recommended revaccinating interval to once every three years for the core vaccines, instead of annually. However, there are still legitimate questions raised over the current practice of giving a dog a booster every third year, as some authorities suggest immunity may be life-long after the puppy vaccines and

---

TITRE TESTS

A titre test is a blood test that measures how much immunity an individual has to a particular disease by checking the level of antibodies in your dog's system. Antibodies are the white blood cells that are important in the immune response, so by measuring them it helps your vet to know whether your dog needs revaccinating or not. However, antibodies are only one component of your dog's immune system; there are many other, less easily measurable, ways in which his body protects itself. Therefore titre test results are not an all-encompassing measure of immunity, they are only part of the picture. Another problem is that if the titre test result shows that your dog requires a booster for one particular disease component only, this may not be possible in practice because most vaccines currently come part and parcel as a multi-agent product.

---

the first annual booster. In fact the latest guidelines (2010) from the World Small Animal Veterinary Association (WSAVA) advised that dogs that had responded to their initial vaccines maintained a solid immunity for many years in the absence of repeat vaccination. One way to help you to assess whether your dog needs his immunity boosting is by having a titre test done.

There are only rarely any immediate side effects of vaccination; these include swelling at the injection site or non-specific signs of tiredness or lethargy for twenty-four hours.

Homeopathic vaccinations

These are homeopathic remedies, called nosodes, made from the infectious agents that we vaccinate dogs against. It is very unfortunate and misleading that they are often termed 'homeopathic vaccinations' – because they are not at all the same as vaccines. Homeopathic nosodes are sometimes given in lieu of vaccinations because they are believed to offer protection against the infectious diseases, without causing any of the adverse reactions associated with conventional vaccines. However, there is currently no reliable evidence to suggest that they offer any protective immunity to your dog at all. Homeopathic nosodes are certainly not a substitute for vaccinations, and homeopathic veterinary surgeons do not support or recommend using them as such.

The holistic approach to vaccination

After weighing up the risks and benefits of vaccinating your dog, the clearest and most sensible solution is to follow the current WSAVA guidelines. These are based on current and scientific knowledge, and state that all puppies should

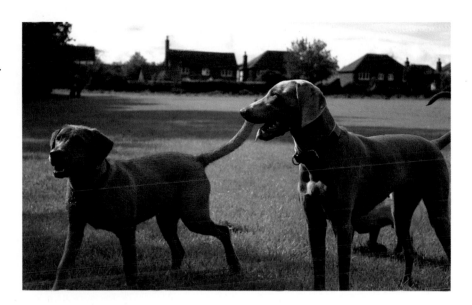

Risk of infection will be different for every dog.

receive an initial primary vaccination with a booster twelve months later. Core vaccinations (covering distemper, parvovirus and hepatitis) are then recommended to be given at intervals of three years or longer, depending on the results of titre tests. Other vaccines, apart from those for the core diseases (commonly for leptospirosis and parainfluenza), may need to be given annually to ensure protection. This protocol ensures that your dog receives the best protection against potentially life-threatening diseases, while minimizing the risk of chronic disease through over-vaccination. However, every dog and every situation is different, and the risks of infection for your dog, in your particular area, may require a different approach. Always discuss vaccinations with your vet, as they will be able to help you evaluate the risk-benefit ratio for your dog and work out the best vaccination protocol for him.

If possible, leave a period of around two weeks between any different vaccines your dog has to have – for example, between his core vaccines and a rabies vaccine. This allows his body more time to respond to them individually, and may reduce the potential for any adverse consequences. In addition, make sure that you only ever have your dog vaccinated when he is in good health, as vaccines target his immune system and will only be advantageous if he is fit and well. Remember that vaccination does not always result in 100 per cent protection from disease and is best used as part of an integrated approach to health for your dog. Finally, in some cases vaccinating your dog will be a legal requirement, such as taking him abroad through the Pet Passport scheme. In this case your dog will need regular rabies vaccinations, as well as his routine annual boosters.

PARASITE CONTROL

The holistic perspective

A parasite is an organism that lives on or in the body of another and feeds off it. All dogs harbour parasites, but not all of them are harmful. From a holistic per-spective, parasite-related health prob-lems stem not from the parasites themselves but from an inability of the host to deal with them effectively. In other words, a healthy dog with a robust immune system should not be adversely affected by most parasites. Health is always fundamentally about maintaining balance, and this means living in balance with a few harmless parasites, however uninviting that sounds. Whether they are the worms that live in your dog's intes-tinal tract, or the fleas that sometimes hop onto him, all these parasites are opportunists, surviving by exploiting a weakness in their host. Therefore your dog will only have a problem with worms, for instance, if he has a poor diet, or if his system is otherwise under stress and cannot cope. Consequently, the holis-tic view of parasites is that they are not the cause of disease; rather, they are a symptom of deeper imbalance within the dog's system. It follows that the most effective and lasting approach to para-sitic infections is to ensure that your dog is as healthy and well nourished as possi-ble. This will make him an uninviting host for the parasites and they will not stay long, soon finding another, weaker dog to colonize. Conventional wormers and flea control treatments should be used when necessary, but not excessively. In healthy dogs, under normal circum-stances, there will be little need to use them often.

WORMING

Why do you need to worm your dog?

Dogs can harbour various kinds of worms, with roundworm and tapeworm being the most common. All dogs are ex-posed to worm infestation at birth and are constantly reinfected throughout their lives. Mostly, they do not cause any noticeable effect on your dog's health. However, worms in significant numbers will sap him of his nutrients and hence be detrimental. Worms are also a potential cause of serious diseases in people.

Roundworms

These are most commonly found in puppies. They are passed on from his mum through the placenta and the milk, even if she was wormed. Roundworms are round white worms like string, which can reach fifteen centimetres in length and live in the intestines. Adult dogs are not usually unduly troubled by round-worms as they are likely to have devel-oped resistance to them.

Tapeworm

Adult dogs get tapeworm through scav-enging and hunting or from contact with other dog's faeces, and also through fleas. Tapeworms live in the intestines, and have a flattened shape like a ribbon, growing up to one metre in length. The presence of tapeworms are actually an indication that the dog's intestinal tract is in an unhealthy state, as they can only hook on and thrive when there are mucus deposits in the intestines in which to shelter. So if your dog suffers with tapeworms, then look to his diet and general state of health, as well as worm-ing him of course.

Lungworm

This parasite has potentially serious consequences for your dog's health, as it affects his respiratory system. Infection is via contact with slugs and snails, as well as through infected dogs' faeces. If your dog is particularly exposed to slugs and snails, have a word with your vet to make

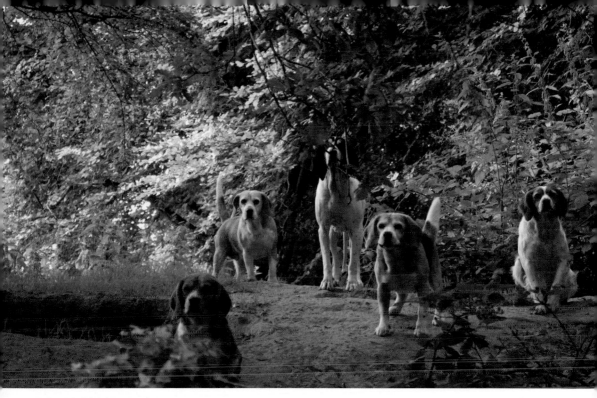

Groups of dogs may need more regular worming.

sure that you are using the correct product to deal with lungworm, as not all wormers will treat for it.

Hookworm and whipworms
These are the only other worms that can potentially affect your dog. However, they are uncommon in this country, and in any case most proprietary wormers will get rid of them

Risk to humans
Most worms that affect your dog can be passed on to humans, usually through contact with dog faeces. Children, pregnant women and people that are immunocompromised are at higher risk. The most significant health risk comes from roundworm, as the larvae can cause serious problems in people, especially children. This is why regular worming, especially of puppies (as they are the most significant carriers of roundworm), is so important. Attention to hygiene after handling your dog, especially for those people such as children and pregnant women who are at highest risk, is another key factor. Finally, picking up after your dog straight away is also important, as this helps to reduce the risk by lowering the environmental worm burden.

Signs of worms
You may not notice any external signs that your dog has worms. However, if he has a significant burden then he may appear in poor condition, with a dull coat and a pot-belly. He may also suffer from digestive upsets such as vomiting or diarrhoea, changes in appetite, and weight loss. If your dog has worms he may lick at or drag his bottom along the ground and have irritation around the anus. Puppies

may also show signs of a bloated abdomen and vomiting. In addition, it is possible for immature stages of some worms to migrate through various other body tissues, and hence affect your dog's liver, kidneys or nervous system. Most worms are microscopic so are not visible to the naked eye, but the tapeworm can be identified like grains of rice at the dog's anus or in his stools.

Treatment

Preventive treatment for worms is recommended, since most dogs harbour them without showing any overt or obvious signs that they have them. Twice yearly is considered sufficient for most adult dogs; however, it may need to be more frequent, depending on the risk factors affecting your dog. For example, worming may be required more often if you walk your dog in an area where there are a lot of other dogs and hence he is at greater risk of reinfestation. Equally, if your dog is at risk from lungworm then monthly worming may be recommended.

Puppies need more frequent worming because they can harbour roundworm passed on to them from their mum. Your vet will be able to weigh and worm him when you take your puppy in for his primary course of vaccines. Puppies are usually wormed every fortnight until they are three months old, and then monthly until they are six months old. From then on follow the recommendations for adult dogs. Flea control is an important part of worm control, because fleas can transmit a type of tapeworm to your dog. While most current worming products available for dogs are considered safe, not all of them are equally effective and some work against certain types of worm and not others. This is why you are recommended to ask your vet's advice about the most appropriate and effective product for your dog. Also, make sure that you weigh him so that you use the correct dose. Wormers are available in a range of different formulation, such as pastes, tablets, powders and liquids or as spot-on preparations that are applied to the skin;

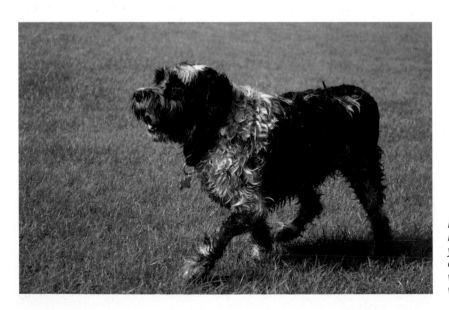

How often you need to worm your dog depends on where you walk him.

choose the easiest dosing method for you and your dog.

Other control measures

It is important to use worming products judiciously because, as with the too frequent use of any of our modern medicines, resistance can build up in the worms that we are trying to eradicate. This has already happened with horses and farm animals where resistance to commonly used worming products is a big problem. A more targeted approach to worming and a good way of reducing unnecessary treatment is to take a faecal sample to your vets for them to perform a test called a faecal egg count. This will alert you as to whether it is necessary to worm your dog. Finally, a simple way of helping keep worm burdens low and hence reduce the risk to both dogs and people is to always pick up your dog's stools and dispose of them properly – 'poop a scoop'. This is a legal requirement in public areas and is also, of course, just part of being a responsible dog owner.

Natural methods

While some of these measures may help to reduce a worm burden, they are often not enough on their own. Indeed, some over-the-counter herbal wormers are excessively harsh on your dog's system. Moreover, there are no homeopathic remedies for 'worming'. This is because homeopathy works by treating the individual rather than the disease. You could use a homeopathic remedy for your dog to boost his general immune system and level of health, but not specifically to kill worms. As regards herbs, there are a few traditional treatments such as garlic, ground or whole pumpkin seeds, grated carrot, shredded coconut, and fennel that

can be added to your dog's diet every so often as a natural worm preventive. Finally, wormwood, as the name suggests, is a folk medicine wormer, but should only be used under professional guidance.

The holistic approach to worming

By keeping your dog in the best of health through his diet and a balanced and stress-free lifestyle, he should not be troubled by worms. For most healthy adult dogs treatment with a broad-spectrum wormer twice a year is sufficient. Using proprietary wormers from the vets is recommended, as these are effective and will usually target all types of worm. Having a faecal egg count carried out on your dog's faeces every so often is a good way of assessing his worm burden and hence the efficacy of your worming programme. Finally, because it was recognized that worms are greatly influenced by the moon, worming of animals was traditionally done at certain times of the month. Worms are known to be more active when the moon is waxing, and so will be less well buried in the host's tissues at this time, and thus easier to get rid of.

FLEAS

Why do you need to use flea treatment?

There are several different species of flea and, paradoxically, the ones that you are more likely to see on your dog are cat fleas, as these are the more common type. Fleas work by injecting anticoagulants into your dog's system and then feeding on his blood. Fleas are a pretty normal parasite of dogs, and usually cause no major health issues at all other than a little irritation every now and again. However, severe flea infestations can be a real problem, and even cause anaemia in very young puppies. Fleas can also carry a type of tapeworm. This is why worming and flea treatment go hand in hand as part of your dog's routine preventive health care. Flea treatment is also especially crucial in dogs that suffer from an allergy to fleas. In such cases, a single bite can trigger a cycle of itching and scratching that will cause great discomfort to the dog and can result in severe skin disease.

Risk to humans

Fleas on your dog can also bite us, usually on the bare skin around the ankles, causing irritation and discomfort. Some people are especially sensitive to flea bites and can be more severely affected, even allergic to them. Fleas do not usually cause further health problems in people. However, don't forget that the flea of the black rat transmitted the bubonic plague, which wiped out a large proportion of the population of England in the fourteenth century.

Signs of fleas

Flea bites can result in considerable annoyance to your dog, causing him to itch, scratch, rub and lick himself all over. Favourite places for fleas are behind your dog's ears, around his tail base, along his back, and in his armpits and groin areas. You may spot a flea if you go through your dog's coat carefully with your fingers and see these small, wingless insects. They are a reddish brown colour and around 2mm long. Sometimes it is tricky to spot fleas like this, so another way of checking for them is to do the following: moisten a piece of white paper and place it beneath your dog, then brush him so that dander falls on the paper. If you see little black specks that turn a red-brown, then that is

positive for fleas, as this occurs when flea droppings, containing blood, dissolve. However, a negative test cannot rule out fleas.

Treatment

Flea treatments for your dog come in various forms; currently the most popular treatments are the 'spot-ons'. These are pipettes filled with an insecticide liquid that is poured onto the back of your dog's neck, between his shoulder blades, usually once a month. This is then absorbed into his skin and sebaceous glands and is thus spread throughout the whole body, killing any fleas as soon as they bite him. Some preparations however, do not kill the flea itself, but otherwise disrupt its breeding and lifecycle. It's a good idea to wear gloves when you are handling these spot-ons and not to touch the treated skin for several hours afterwards. Flea collars, powders, sprays and tablets are other methods of flea control for your dog, and will have varying efficacy depending on their active constituents. Your vet will be able to advise on a suitable treatment and show you how to use it. The most common reasons that flea treatments do not work are if they contain ineffective ingredients, are incorrectly applied or administered, or if not all pets in the household are treated.

Environmental control measures

Treating your dog is just one part on an overall strategy of flea control. Ninety per cent of the flea's lifecycle, the egg, pupae and larval stages, takes place away from your dog, so it's easy to see why environmental measures are the mainstay of effective flea control. These immature stages of the flea will be present in your dog's home environment, in his bedding, on your carpets and soft furnishings and in any nooks and crannies where the conditions are right for them. Their whole lifecycle, from egg to adult, takes anything between two weeks and eight months. Fleas thrive in warm, humid conditions, and do less well in extremes of temperature and in the dry. This is why, although they can be a problem all year round, fleas are usually more of an issue in the spring and autumn when the conditions are most favourable for them. In addition, fleas can stay dormant in the environment for many months, waiting for ambient conditions that will allow them to re-emerge. So if you move into a new home where the previous residents had pets, be extra vigilant in cleaning before you introduce your dog. The simplest means of getting rid of flea larvae, pupae and eggs from your home is to vacuum regularly and wash your dog's bedding every few weeks on a hot cycle. If you have carpets then steam cleaning them is also recommended. Bear in mind that wooden and laminate floors are a much less flea-friendly environments. There are also various household sprays that have active ingredients to control the flea lifecycle. These will usually be chemical-based, but there are more natural products available that use mechanical means of disrupting fleas. Finally, don't forget that every time your dog comes into contact with other dogs, or cats, he can potentially pick up a new crop of fleas, which he can then bring back into the house and so start off the whole flea cycle all over again. This is why flea prevention is an ongoing process.

Natural methods
Natural methods are usually only suitable as flea repellents, rather than as actual means of eliminating them. Where there are significant infestations of fleas, or if your dog has a flea allergy, then conventional treatments such as the spot-ons will usually be called for. However, in all other situations natural methods of flea prevention can play an important role in helping you to reduce your reliance on chemical means, and help your dog to resist fleas naturally. These include, first and foremost, simply using a flea comb on your dog. These have tines that are so fine that they will mechanically rid your dog's coat of the fleas quickly and efficiently. Bathing him and making a good lather also helps to kill any fleas, but won't be a sufficient flea prevention measure on its own. If you are using a specific anti-flea shampoo, be aware that pennyroyal, although it is well known as a flea-repellent herb and hence is present in many shampoos and rinses, contains volatile oils that can be highly toxic to dogs. A cumulative risk will therefore exist for dogs that lick off these topical preparations, so it is best avoided. If you are opting for using an herbal flea-repellent for your dog, either as a rinse for his coat or as a dried herb sprinkled on his bed, be aware that the herbs need to be fresh otherwise they will have lost their potency. Pyrethrum is derived from chrysanthemum flowers and is one of nature's best insecticides. Both natural and synthetic versions of this compound are widely used as the active constituent in many flea products. Adding a little fresh garlic to your dog's diet every so often can also act as a natural flea-repellent. It should not, however, be fed in quantities that cause any garlic odour to exude from his skin, as it will be potentially toxic at such high strengths. Brewer's yeast is another dietary supplement that is sometimes cited as having flea-repellent function. This is debatable, however, and many dogs have sensitivi-

ties to it. Other so-called natural approaches to flea control in the home include borax powders and diatomaceous earth. However, these should be avoided too, since borax can be toxic and diatomaceous earth can cause irritation if inhaled. Electronic flea-collars are not recommended either because, as well as being ineffective, the electromagnetic signals may interfere with the dog's own energy systems.

The holistic approach to flea treatment

As with the internal parasites, a few fleas are to be expected, as your dog can pick them up whenever he goes out or meets another dog, even if your home is flea-free. By feeding your dog well, and thereby ensuring that he has a robust immune system and a shiny coat rich in natural oils, you will be preventing him from being unduly affected by fleas. In addition to these overall health and dietary means, using natural methods of flea prevention, such as regular flea combing, herbal rinses, and the addition of garlic in the diet, alongside rigorous vacuuming, should be enough in most cases. However, if fleas are still a problem, or if your dog has a particular sensi-

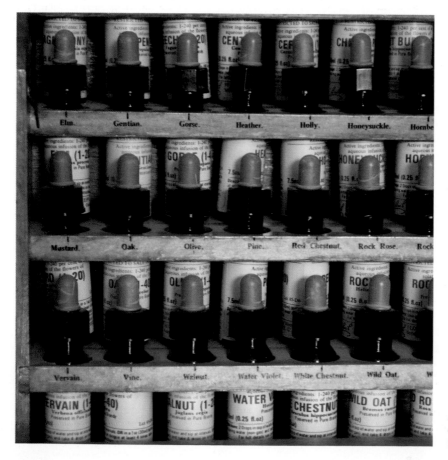

Natural methods can be effective flea-repellents.

tivity to them, then the judicious use of insecticide spot-ons is justified. This helps to break the flea lifecycle and to get on top of the situation before a few fleas rapidly become a lot of fleas. But it's as well to try and use these insecticides as little as possible, because the chemicals in most flea treatments will eventually end up reaching waterways and landfill sites and thus affecting the environment. Indeed, the class of insecticides widely blamed for the recent mass disappearance of the honeybee is in fact the active constituent in the most commonly used spot-on flea treatments. If these products can harm fleas and bees, we should question what the long term consequences of monthly applications to your dog could be.

NEUTERING

What is neutering?

Neutering is the general term used to describe 'de-sexing' an animal; it means the same as spaying in females and castrating in males. Spaying is an operation to remove the entire female reproductive tract, similar to an ovariohysterectomy in women. Castration is the removal of the testes. Both operations are performed under general anaesthesia and, although major operations, are procedures that your vet will be doing every day. In most cases your dog will only be kept in the veterinary hospital for the day, able to go home in the evening. They will have to return to the surgery for post-operative checks and sometimes for the removal of stitches. It will be expected that you keep your dog quiet for around one or two weeks following their surgery; this is especially important for bitches. The most important reason for having your dog neutered is so that they can't have puppies. This is a

responsible choice given the number of abandoned and unwanted dogs that already need homes. However, it is important to weigh up the positive as well as the negative aspects of neutering before making the decision for your dog.

Why neuter dogs?

There are no valid medical reasons to routinely castrate every male dog; it depends on the individual and the situation.

Roaming after bitches

If he is prone to going off after bitches on heat then it is common to have your dog castrated to try and prevent such behaviour. With lower testosterone levels he should have less urge to stray.

Behaviour problems

This is not a reason to castrate your dog. Behaviour-related problems are down to the individual dog and how they have been socialized and what they have learnt through their past experiences; they are not related to the sex of the dog. In fact recent studies have shown that neutered dogs are actually more likely to suffer from fearful aggression and other behaviour problems than those that are left entire.

For medical reasons

Castration may be part of the recommended treatment for dogs suffering from prostatic or testicular disease, for example. It is also important that your dog is castrated if he has a retained testicle.

Why neuter bitches?

No puppies and no seasons

A bitch is neutered to stop her having puppies. This is advantageous because it means you won't be adding to the vast number of unwanted dogs that already need homes. Remember that if she does have puppies you will need to find homes for them all, as well as cover the extra costs involved in breeding. Having your bitch neutered also means that she won't come into season twice a year. This is an advantage because a bitch in season can be messy to have around the house, as she will be dripping blood for a few days. If you have your bitch neutered it also means that you won't have to worry about taking her out for walks and fending off unwanted male dogs twice a year when she is in season. Therefore a neutered bitch can be easier to manage from a practical point of view.

For health reasons
Statistics show that neutering a bitch before her first season reduces the risk of her developing mammary tumours in later life, and can increase her life expectancy. Another advantage of neutering her is that it will prevent her from getting an infection in her womb, a pyometra, a condition that can affect older bitches.

The optimum age to neuter
For male dogs, castration is usually done at about six months of age. For bitches, however, the situation is less clear-cut. While early neutering is advocated as providing better protection against mammary tumours, it is also considered to be a risk factor for the development of incontinence. Incontinence can occur in a small percentage of neutered bitches, usually in medium and large breeds. It is thought to be a consequence of the neck of the bladder not remaining tight, possibly due to the change in hormone levels or because of mechanical changes in the female tract as a result of neutering. It is thought that by allowing the bitch to have one season before she is neutered the risk of incontinence is reduced, so this is the usual advice for medium and larger breed bitches. It is also widely agreed that for the overall mental and emotional, as well as the physical, development of a bitch, she should be allowed to have at least one season. The decision is therefore always a tricky one, so it will be worthwhile talking it through with your vet and finding out the best option for your particular bitch. Bitches usually have their first season at around six months, but this can vary and be much later in some individuals.

Neutering and obesity
A neutered dog usually has a slightly lower metabolic rate, and may have a keener interest in food, than an entire dog. Both of these situations can lead to dogs of either sex gaining weight after neutering. However, this situation can be avoided by altering your dog's diet to match his lower energy requirements, and of course by simply not overfeeding him

Neutering and behaviour changes
The widely held view that neutered dogs are better behaved and easier to live with is not based on fact. The reality is that your dog's behaviour is down to his socialization as a puppy, and his training and learning experiences throughout his life, not to do with what sex he is or whether he is neutered. In fact, recent reports point to greater behaviour problems in neutered pets. Other research showed less age-related cognitive impairment in entire males than in their neutered counterparts.

The holistic approach to neutering
According to homeopathic and other

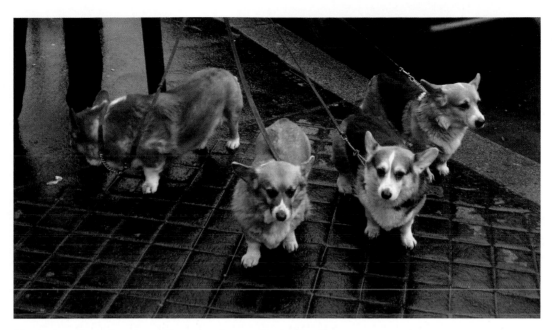

Neutering doesn't necessarily make dogs easier to handle.

holistic philosophies, removing an entire organ system has a fundamental knock-on effect on the rest of the body. This is because its method of 'rebalancing' itself in the face of disease has been altered. This may sound nonsensical, and it would be if you viewed the reproductive tract in isolation, just as a means of producing offspring. However, from the holistic or whole body perspective the reproductive tract has a more diverse role in maintaining health. So although in this respect neutering is not natural, it can also be argued that keeping your dog entire without allowing him to breed is equally unnatural. Having him neutered will mean that your dog will not be frustrated by experiencing hormonal impulses that he is not allowed to fulfil. Of course every dog is different, and for those that have few sexual urges remaining entire and not breeding will be of little consequence

to them. Ultimately, you can only decide whether to have your dog neutered after weighing up all the pros and cons and after talking it through with your vet.

TAKING YOUR DOG ABROAD

The European Pet Passport (EU Pet Passport) allows for qualifying dogs to cross borders and move around freely within Europe. The Pet Travel Scheme (PETS) provides for qualifying dogs to travel to and from the UK from certain listed countries without undergoing quarantine. In order to qualify, your dog must have been microchipped and have had a rabies vaccination and a blood test, in that order. It is a fairly expensive and lengthy process and must be carried out by an approved veterinary surgeon. Be aware that there is a six-month wait from the date of the satisfactory blood sample before you can bring your dog back into the country. Since the blood test is usually done between two and four weeks after your dog's rabies vaccination, the whole process takes at least eight months. Therefore you need to plan well ahead if you are considering taking your dog away on holiday with you. In addition, between twenty-four and forty-eight hours before re-entering the country, your dog will have to be checked by a vet. He will need to have a satisfactory health check and has to be treated for ticks and worms using approved medications. In addition, you will need to travel using an approved transport company and use an approved route. Your dog's subsequent rabies boosters need to be done according to the exact date they are due, usually once every two years. Going overdue by even one day means restarting the whole process. The participating countries and exact details of these schemes are subject to change, so always get up-to-date information from DEFRA before planning your trip.

Disease risk

It is also important to remember that when he is abroad, especially in warmer climes, your dog may be exposed to diseases that we do not have in this country. Some of these can be fatal, or at least cause serious illness, and may also be transmissible to people. One example of this is the processional caterpillars of southern France, Spain and other parts of the Mediterranean. These caterpillars, which move along joined together in chains, are covered in fine hairs containing a toxin that can cause severe allergic reactions. Dogs that sniff or touch them may, in severe cases, end up losing parts of their tongue – or indeed, it can even be fatal. Heartworm is another parasitic disease that we thankfully don't have in this country at present. It is carried by mosquitoes and occurs in warmer countries, including the USA. Hence for dogs that are taken abroad to warmer climes, preventive heartworm treatment is important. If that isn't enough to put you off, also consider how different climates and long journeys may affect your dog. He may not be as comfortable in the heat as you are, especially if he is longcoated or elderly. For all of these reasons it is important to think very carefully about whether it is in your dog's best interests to take him on holiday with you.

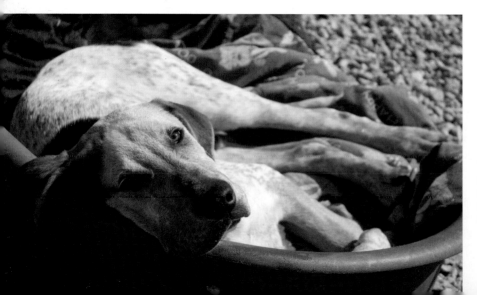

Your dog may be more comfortable staying at home.

6 DIET AND NUTRITION

Let your food be your medicine, and let medicine be your food.

Hippocrates

A nutritious diet is the foundation of good health, without which truly 'holistic' care will not be possible. Therefore the importance of your dog's daily diet cannot be underestimated. You need to know that what you are feeding him is providing your dog with all the building blocks his body needs in order to stay fit and healthy. This chapter introduces the concept of a complete and balanced diet. It also explains how the canine digestive system works, and hence the best way to feed your dog. Finally, by taking a look at how mass-produced dog foods are manufactured, you will be able to decide whether this is the most nutritious and appropriate way to feed him.

A BALANCED DIET

A balanced diet will contain all the key nutrients in the correct proportions to allow your dog to be active and healthy. His individual dietary needs will depend on his age, state of health and level of activity. Therefore there is no single diet that will suit every dog. Ideally his daily rations will contain fresh lean meat, some lightly cooked wholegrain cereals and

A nutritious diet is the foundation of good health.

vegetables, and a little oil and fruits. This will provide your dog with an optimum balance of the seven nutrients vital for life: protein, fats, carbohydrates, fibre, vitamins, minerals and water. These are the building blocks for each and every

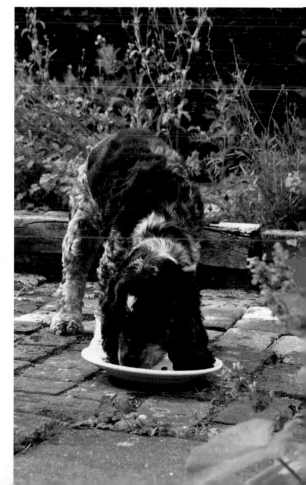

cell in his body. They play an important role in maintenance as well as repair, keeping your dog physically and mentally strong and balanced. Your dog's food is also the fuel that keeps him active and drives all his bodily functions. Variety is another key to a balanced diet. Using foods that are in season and tailoring your dog's diet to his individual needs are fundamental to the philosophy of using foods for health and healing. As well as what you feed him, you also need to consider how much to feed your dog every day. With obesity so commonplace, this is important. Remember that feeding guidelines on labels, or other recommendations such as diet sheets or recipes, will be for the average dog of a given size or weight. They do not take account of individual needs such as age, breed, metabolism, activity level and state of health. Each of these factors will play a role in how much you need to feed your dog, which may well vary from the average. You may need to seek advice about feed-

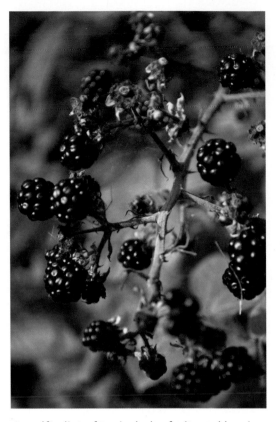

A wolf's diet often includes fruits and berries.

OBESITY

Recent reports suggest that one in four dogs in the UK is obese. The reasons, in the vast majority of cases, are the same as for obese humans: eating too much, or the wrong type of food, and not getting enough exercise. It will come as no surprise to learn that these dogs are putting greater strain on their hearts and joints and are more likely to be affected by chronic illness in later life. Prevent your dog from becoming overweight in the first place by giving him plenty of regular exercise and feeding him a healthy diet.

ing your dog in particular circumstances such as pregnancy, or for greater or reduced levels of activity.

THE CANINE DIGESTIVE SYSTEM

In order to find out what we should feed our domestic dogs, we need to go back and look at the diet of their closest wild ancestor, the wolf.

The wolf's diet

Wolves are flexible, opportunistic predators. Their prey is largely made up of herbivores such as rabbits, antelope or deer, depending on where they live and the time of year. Not only are wolves predators, they are also scavengers, eating whatever is most easily available to them. The term carnivore refers to species that obtain most of their nutrition through eating meat. Even though wolves are carnivores, and there is no doubt that they do acquire a large percentage of their food from prey, they are not exclusively meat eaters. In fact, a wolf's diet commonly includes a variety of fruits, nuts and other plant foods.

Carnivore and scavenger

Dogs are carnivores and scavengers too, having been domesticated from wolves over many thousands of years. Since the early days of domestication, man used dogs to help him hunt and to guard his settlements. He would doubtless have fed his new companion by throwing him carcasses and other leftovers from the kill. Throughout this time these newly domesticated dogs would also have had access to the remains of man's cooked food. This, together with the stomach contents of the prey they ate, would have provided dogs with the cereal and other vegetable parts of their diets. They augmented this by grazing on the various grasses, berries and mosses that they sought out for themselves. Hence, it is clear that by feeding our modern-day dogs a diet based on raw meat and bones, along with some cooked wholegrain cereals and liquidized veg, we can closely mirror that of their ancestors.

Dogs are often classified as omnivores, able to survive on a diet of vegetables or meats. Indeed, it was this flexibility in their digestive ability that was one of their greatest strengths in evolution: having a dentition that was adapted to either meat or plant-based foodstuffs, whichever was more abundant. Dogs

have teeth, the carnassials, that are both cutting and shearing for tearing meat, which gives them the carnivore tag. But they also have a full set of snatching incisors and grinding molars, for the vegetable matter. However, it is widely acknowledged that dogs are better classified as facultative carnivores. In other words, they do much better when fed a meat-rich diet. By observing their natural feeding preferences, and on further examination of their digestive systems, there is no question that dogs were designed to eat meat and bones. Another adaptation from dog's scavenging past is their strong stomach acid, relatively short intestinal tract, and fast food transit time. These, among other features of their digestion, helped dogs to cope with their diet of often rotten and rancid foods. Finally, it is also interesting to consider how wild dogs feed themselves. They scavenge and eat whatever is available, so that their diet does not consist of daily 'balanced' meals. Instead it is described as being 'balanced over time', which means that it is balanced, but not in every meal. Thus they get all the nutrition they need over several days, eating what they find and following their instincts to seek out the nutrients they are lacking. Of course this would not be a successful way of managing the nutritional requirements of most of our pet dogs, but it is nonetheless a thought-provoking concept in the evolution of canine nutrition.

FEEDING YOUR DOG

You can feed your dog easily and well by giving him a diet based on the following foods: raw meaty bones, organ meat, liquidized raw or lightly cooked seasonal vegetables, a little oil and some cooked

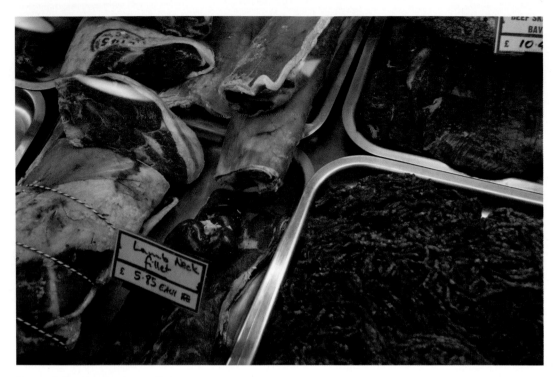

Dogs thrive on a meaty diet.

wholegrains such as oats, barley or rice. Feeding a variety of different types of meat, vegetables and grains helps to ensure that your dog gets the full quota of nutrients he needs. Using organically certified meat means that as well as being free from antibiotic and chemical residues it will have come from farms practising higher animal welfare. If you are new to cooking for or preparing your dog's meals yourself, then it is advisable to talk to your vet as well as the growing number of dog owners turning to this way of feeding. They will be able to give you practical advice, such as the amounts to feed, and which local butchers to use. Don't forget that although this way of feeding you dog is not difficult and has enormous health benefits, it still requires more time and commitment that simply opening a can or a bag of kibble. An alternative to the home-cooked diet is to choose a diet made by one of the small-scale producers that emulate the 'home-cooked' approach.

The BARF Diet

This way of feeding your dog is sometimes called the BARF diet, which stands for 'Bones As Raw Food' or 'Biologically Appropriate Raw Food'. Fundamentally this diet consists of feeding both raw meat and raw bones (chicken wings are commonly used). Usually some raw vegetables and fruits are added to it, after pureeing or liquidising. Dogs are generally very healthy on this diet, with glossy coats, shiny white teeth and a spring in their step. This is in part due to the raw nature of the diet, and because it is so closely matched to that of your dog's wolf ancestors. It has not undergone any cooking or processing whatsoever, so the food has not lost any of its nutritional value or its important digestive enzymes. This makes it easier for your dog to digest, and is why raw food is full of vitality. By so closely matching the wolf's diet, dogs can thrive on this way of feeding as it suits their digestive system, and is what they were designed to eat. Raw bones keep your dog's teeth clean and tartar-free and, unlike cooked bones, they are unlikely to splinter as he gnaws them. One of the oft-cited risks of a raw meat diet is that of the food poisoning bugs salmonella and E. coli. They are undeniably a cause for concern with this way of feeding. However, these infections are actually more of a worry for your own health than for that of your dog, since he has a very acidic stomach to help him cope with any nasty bacteria, and you don't. To reduce the risks, be careful of where you source the meat and be vigilantly hygienic when it comes to preparation and feeding. If you like the sound of this diet, read up on it, seek expert advice, and make up your own mind. To help take the hard work out of it there are now even companies that will prepare raw meat diets for your dog in frozen meal-sized portions and deliver them to your door.

Food therapy

In Traditional Chinese Medicine foods are commonly used to rebalance energy and promote healing. Each food is linked to a particular direction, flavour, organ system and temperature, such that each patient will be prescribed a diet based on their

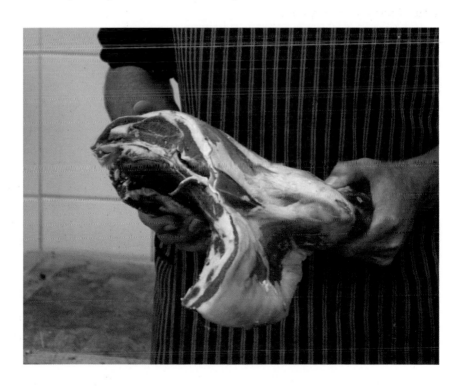

The BARF diet is popular.

VEGETARIAN DIETS

Dogs are facultative carnivores, which means that although they can in theory survive on a meat-free diet, it is not what they would eat given the choice. Remember that a dog's digestive system was designed for a meat-based diet and that this is what the species, as a whole, prefers to eat. If you do decide to go ahead and feed a vegetarian diet to your dog, it is much easier and more sensible to choose one of the propri-etary vegetarian dog foods than to attempt home cooking. These will have been specifically formulated to meet prescribed nutritional criteria using all animal-free ingredients.

own particular symptoms. Much Western herbal medicine has for centuries also relied on the energetic qualities of herbs and foodstuffs to perform particular actions in the body and to restore health. Therefore, by having an understanding of the basic properties of some of the key constituents of the diet, you can help support your dog's system with healing foods. However, by simply feeding him meat and vegetables that are in season, you are already practising very simple food therapy.

THE PET FOOD INDUSTRY

The simplicity of feeding your dog meat, cereal and some vegetables is now a global industry. In 2008 the value of the UK pet food industry alone was just under two billion pounds. Commercially produced dog foods, usually as cans of meat or bags of dry food, known as kibble, have been a booming industry since after World War II, when mass production first began. It quickly took off as people saw how easily they could feed their dogs 'all in one' meals from a can. Before this they would have fed them raw or cooked meat and vegetables, together with scraps from the table. It was great for the manufacturers too; they were suddenly able to make their leftover by-products into saleable goods. Of course, with such a huge industry, there is now a wide variation in the way that dog food is manufactured commer-cially. This ranges from the small 'kitchen-table' producers to the mass-market industry where, every second, millions of cans run off production lines all over the world. In terms of nutritional value and health-giving properties, the differences

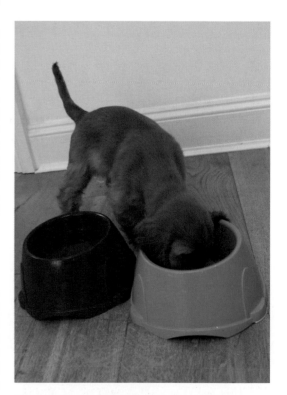

Most dogs are fed mass-produced food.

are as vast as the scale and method of manufacture. With just a handful of global conglomerates currently manufacturing over three-quarters of the dog food available in the UK, the vast majority of dogs are still fed on the mass-produced diets outlined here.

What goes into the can?

Firstly, let's look at the meat that goes into dog food. The majority is labelled as 'meat and animal derivatives'. According to animal feed legislation, this is meat that is surplus to human consumption or not normally consumed by people in this country, but is passed as being fit for human consumption. This information would probably lead you to understand that it is just leftover meat, perfectly edible to us, but which we either have too much of, or we don't usually consume. What you wouldn't imagine is that this meat, classified as 'animal by-products', is stuff that we would never even contemplate eating; we are talking about feathers, hair, hooves, eyes, you name it. This is why the term 'fit for human consumption' in the original statement is misleading. Because by 'fit' it means that the material is free of transmissible diseases and does not derive from dead or dying animals. These 'meat and animal derivatives' need to then somehow end up as tasty dog food. This is usually done via a process of slow cooking called rendering. Rendered meat can be from any source, any animal, and almost any part of it; the label will just say 'meat and bone meal', or 'meat and animal derivatives'. Manufacturers must of course ensure that their foods are 'complete and balanced'. How they manage to do this, however, can be quite extraordinary. For example, grains, such as corn or rice, are used as cheap sources of protein and fillers, in place of meat. Of course being so high in grains, these processed diets do not mirror the natural canine diet and hence can be difficult for dogs to digest. Many believe that this is largely to blame for the increasing number of dogs suffering from wheat intolerances and dietary sensitivities. Moreover, wheat gluten and other protein gels are sometimes used in wet dog foods to create artificial 'meaty chunks' and give the food a texture that helps it look like real meat.

The next disappointment is the 'derivatives of vegetable origin'. This translates as the green leafy vegetables that you think have gone into the bag or can, and indeed may have featured on the label. These have undergone a similar fate to the meat and are just reprocessed leftovers. When these meat and vegetable derivatives have been mixed together, the next step in making dry dog food is to put it through a pressure steamer to dehydrate it and make it into biscuits. These will then be sprayed with emulsifiers, fats and other additives and preservatives to prolong their shelf life and make them tasty. The vitamins and minerals are also usually added back to the meat at this point, as all the naturally occurring goodness will have been lost through the lengthy, high-temperature industrial processing. There is also the addition of artificial additives that help to preserve the food, make it look nice, colourful and healthy, and make sure your dog will love it. The food for sale in veterinary practices often makes up a significant part of their income, and the vast majority of this is made by the huge multinationals that produce most of the pet food worldwide. It's just like it is in the human food chain: a few big players corner the market and with their vast advertising budgets make their foods

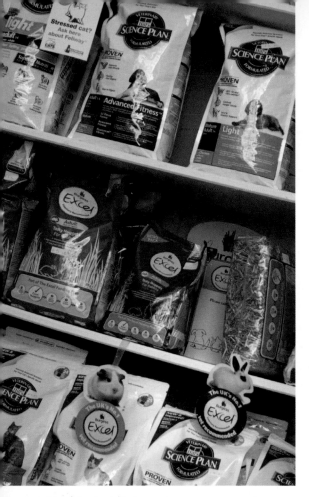

Mass-produced diets.

appear fantastic for your dog. We've all seen those TV adverts of a dog bouncing through the fields on his way home for a slap-up meal of canned food.

'Natural' commercial diets

This is a burgeoning area of the dog food market. With growing awareness of some of the shortcomings of mass-produced foods, there is a demand for commercial diets that are more 'natural' and wholesome. Although this is good news, not all such diets have an equally good provenance. It's often necessary to distinguish those manufacturers that have a genuine interest in a 'natural' approach to nutri-tion from those that are just jumping on the latest bandwagon. Be aware that most of the mass-producers have now brought out their own 'natural' ranges too. So although such descriptions as 'wholesome', 'traditional', 'as nature intended' and 'real' can be, and to some extent should be, dismissed as woolly, labelling law does hold some weight. It directs that any food using the above descriptions pertaining to a natural provenance should be additive-free and have a low-impact, smaller-scale and traditional manufacture and preservation process. In addition, the raw ingredients in dog foods that are described as in any way 'natural' should be in the can, or bag, as nature intended. That is to say if it contains lamb or chicken, these should be the actual meat, rather than derivatives or by-products, and any grains should be wholegrain and not refined or milled. It is also assumed that these foods will have been processed by slow cooking and preserved using natural preservatives. This way the ingredients retain their innate nutritional qualities and can be digested and used by the body in a gentle manner, as they should be. Un-fortunately, however, clever marketing and ambiguous wording and packaging can still easily mislead the unwary cus-tomer. This is where it really pays to do your homework. In fact, there are cur-rently only two criteria pertaining to natural pet foods where stringent regula-tions apply. These are 'organic' and 'holis-tic', and even these words are widely bandied about and misused, so to be certain of specific minimum standards you must make sure that the bag or can is actually stamped with the symbol of a recognized certification body. In the UK these are most often the Soil Association or the Organic Farmers and Growers

Find out what's in your dog's food.

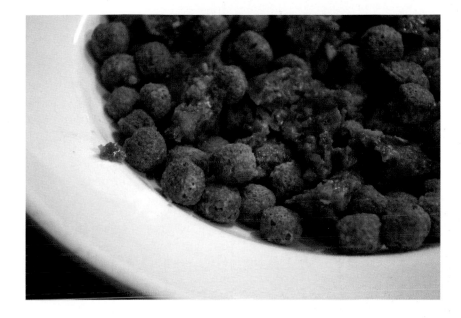

Association. Certified organic dog food will therefore contain meat derived from higher welfare farms where unnecessary antibiotics and growth promoters will not have been used. Similarly, the vegetables and fruits will have been grown without the use of synthetic fertilizers and will be free of genetically modified organisms. There is only one 'certified holistic' regulatory body, namely the British Association of Holistic Nutrition and Medicine. This has a code of ethics and principles that are similar to those of the organic movement but with the added dimension that the foods used should be appropriate for the species in question. Holistic certified foods should therefore contain unprocessed raw ingredients derived from plant and animal sources in their natural state. Being appropriate means that the food will reflect as much as possible the natural diet of the dog's wild ancestor, so will therefore be most easily digestible and optimally nutritious for them.

Choosing a commercial diet

If you have decided that this is going to be the best way to feed your dog, choosing which brand and type of commercial food is best for him needs a little homework. If you are looking at the food in the shop, read the label carefully, but also try and have a look at the food itself. Ask to see an open bag or can, or better still arrange to take a sample home. Have a close look, smell and feel of the food when you put it out into your dog's bowl. Do your homework about the company that makes it and arm yourself with enough information so that you know exactly what has gone into your chosen dog food. Getting your dog to try it is all well and good, but as we know dogs are fairly indiscriminate and will usually wolf down anything. This is why it lies with us as owners to ensure that what we put down for our dogs to eat is healthy and nutritious. Where is the meat sourced? What grains are in it and how are they cooked? How is the food preserved?

What is the company's stance on animal testing? A list of approved manufacturers that adhere to certain criteria with regard to animal testing can be obtained via the organization People for the Ethical Treatment of Animals (PETA). Any ethical, caring dog food company will value their customers and be happy to answer all your questions.

THE QI IN FOOD

A final thought from the ancient Chinese philosophers, who believed that vital energy, Qi, comes from the food that we eat (they call it 'Gu Qi'). This energy originates in the raw ingredient, because every living thing has its own energy, but is then altered during the cooking or manufacturing process. It follows that the lovingly home-produced meal will have so much more healing and health-giving substance to it, better 'qi', than the machine-made pellet. This is another reason why meat from factory-farmed animals will not be providing your dog with 'good energy', as we are all well aware of how these animals are treated. Therefore, from the energetic perspective, mass-produced processed food is both lacking in vitality and perhaps even contains 'bad' energy, or bad karma. This is an aspect of food and nutrition that is undoubtedly a far cry from the analytical and material, but it is one of the foundations of Traditional Chinese Medicine and has been a recipe for health for over 4,000 years.

UNDERSTANDING THE LABEL

The Food Standards Agency is responsible for the labelling of farm animal food because it is part of the human food chain. Pet food, however, has far less information on its labels, and is under the jurisdiction of local Trading Standards. So while you can find out the details of what goes into a cow's food, the same is not true for that of your dog. However, regulations do require there to be a statutory statement on every label on every commercially available dog food. It must contain the following obligatory declarations.

Product description This will indicate whether it is a 'complete' food, or a 'complementary' food (such as treats or a mixer); which species it is for; and directions for feeding.

Typical analysis The percentage of the following must be listed: proteins, oils and fats, fibre, moisture content (if it is over 14 per cent), and finally ash (ash represents the mineral content of the food, and is determined by burning the product, hence it is termed ash content).

Ingredients list Every ingredient must be listed, in descending order by amount. They can either be indicated by their category, such as 'meat and animal derivatives' or 'cereal', or by their own individual names; this is up to the manufacturer.

Additives If preservatives, antioxidants or colours have been added to the product, their presence has to be declared by using the category or chemical name of the additive. However, the term 'EC permitted additives' contains a possible 4,000 chemicals, many of which have been banned from human foods.

Vitamins If vitamins A, D or E have been added, their presence and level has to be declared. The level must include the quantity naturally present in the food.

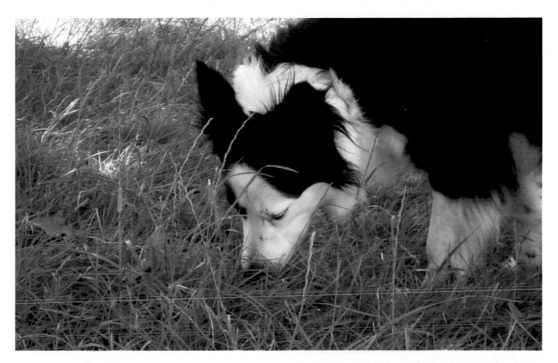

Dogs naturally chew grass to cleanse their digestive systems.

Best before date After this date the product may start to deteriorate.

Net weight This is the weight of the actual food, excluding the packaging.

Name and address The manufacturer, packer, importer, seller or distributor.

MEALTIMES

How often you need to feed your dog depends on his digestion, metabolism and also on your own routine and lifestyle. A twice-daily meal, with the second one not being too late in the day is the most usual feeding regime; after all, carnivores usually hunt at dawn and dusk. However, every dog is different;

ADDITIVES

It is hardly surprising that hyperactivity and other behaviour problems are so often linked to diet. Simply by changing to a food that is additive-free will usually make the world of difference to your dog. These additives are the 'necessary evils' of the mass-manufacturing process. They ensure that the food ends up being tasty, looking appetizing and able to stay fresh for months or years. They include emulsifiers, lubricants, anti-caking agents, drying agents, thickeners, colourings, sweeteners, animal digest, flavourings, texturizers and grease; the list goes on. In addition to the harmful effects of these additives by themselves, when added together the effect is a relatively unknown.

some prefer their main, or only, meal in the morning while others don't like to eat anything until mid-afternoon. You will need to learn your own dog's preferences by trial and error. Puppies, of course, do need small meals and frequent feeding. It is always good practice to remove any uneaten food and not to leave food down for your dog all the time.

Manners and training mustn't be forgotten when it comes to mealtimes. Basic ground rules include never feeding your dog from the table or allowing him to beg for food. Regular mealtimes are also important for dogs, as is feeding them in the same place. In TCM the spleen, an Earth organ, is crucial to the digestive processes, and is very sensitive to and easily upset by changes in routine. So if you have a dog that is of an 'Earth' constitution (see Chapter 2), their digestion may be more prone to upset by

changes of routine, resulting in problems such as loose stools. As well as regularity, calm and quiet can be thought of as the emotional 'seasoning' for a healthy digestive process, so having a quiet place for your dog to eat is one of the best routines to try and establish. If you have more than one dog, feeding time can be quite stressful, especially if one dog eats faster than the other and there is competition over the food. This is why in some cases it is better to feed your dogs in separate rooms.

If you are changing your dog's diet, always do so slowly over a few weeks by gradually substituting the old food with the new. In addition, make sure that your dog's food bowl is not plastic, because used day after day, petrochemicals may leach out into the food. Ceramic bowls are usually best, as stainless steel or metal bowls can be noisy. If your dog is a fussy

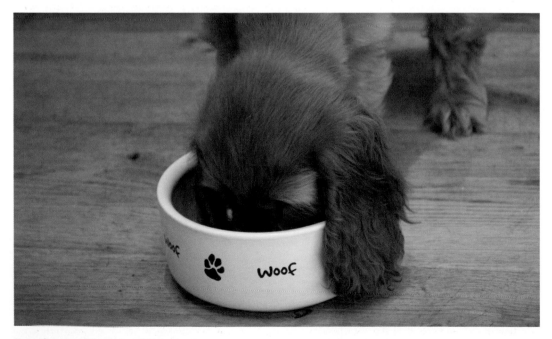

Regular mealtimes are important.

WATER

Having fresh water available to your dog at all times is vital. Bottled water has been linked to health concerns associated with the leaching of plastics, and with environmental damage. Therefore using filtered water is a good option. You may have noticed that your dog prefers to drink from puddles and buckets outside; this may be because rainwater is free of the chemicals found in tap water, but it does carry its own risks such as bacterial infection. Offer water in a clean ceramic bowl and change it at least daily, ensuring that it is well filled. Watch out that your dog has always got access to his water bowl. If necessary, have one in different rooms at home, for instance if he is less mobile or elderly. Don't forget to carry fresh drinking water for your dog when you are travelling, either in the car or even just on a walk.

eater, it may help to try feeding him from a range of different dishes to see whether he prefers one of a certain size, height or type. He may also prefer to be fed somewhere quiet, on his own.

Your dog should, whenever possible, be able to have his food without it being adulterated. This usually means without the addition of medications or similar. Therefore, unless it is absolutely essential that a medicine is given as part of a full meal (ask your vet if this is the case), it is better to give your dog any medicine he may need in a little separate food, or with a treat. This is because by adding medicine to your dog's food you are inadvertently compromising his basic right to his food, as he will be faced with having to eat it with the medicine or to go without. This is obviously not a fair choice for him, and may also pave the way for a dog to become a fussy eater.

DISCUSSION

'You are what you eat.' Therefore however you choose to feed your dog, it is the quality of the ingredients and making sure that he has a diet that is balanced and appropriate for his digestive system that is crucial. But it's also important to assess whether what you are feeding him actually suits your dog's individual constitution and condition. Not every way of feeding, every recipe or every brand of food brings out the best in every dog, because of individual differences relating to age, breed, metabolic rate and constitutional factors. Your dog needs to enjoy his food. Mealtimes should be nourishing for his spirit and mind, as well as for his body. The Ayurvedic and the Ancient Chinese say that you have to eat right for your 'body-type' and for the season, so don't forget that this applies to your dog too. To assess whether your dog's diet suits him, pay attention to how he looks and acts. How much energy does he have? How does he behave? What is his coat like? Is it shiny and glossy or dry and dull? How are his stools? How much water does he drink? Is his weight stable? How do his teeth look? Is he suffering from tartar build-up and sore gums? Is he in optimum health? Or is he suffering from chronic health issues? The answers to each of these questions will be key pointers in helping you to decide whether your dog's diet is the best for him. Diet is the cornerstone of health and therefore needs to be the first thing that you address in any aspect of basic health care or healing.

7 SUPPLEMENTS FOR HEALTH

Supplements are used to promote health and prevent disease. They are the most rapidly evolving area of the pet health care market. This chapter introduces the most commonly used supplements for dogs, explaining what they are used for and how they work. In simple terms these are products derived from natural substances that have been refined, concentrated, and sometimes adapted, to provide a specific health-giving effect. They are usually given to your dog daily with food in the form of powders, tablets, capsules or liquids. 'Nutraceuticals' was coined as a marketing term to make supplements sound more akin to 'pharmaceuticals', and hence more effective. While it is excellent news that there are so many dog health products out there, they can vary widely in terms of quality and effectiveness, which can sometimes make choosing the right one difficult. This chapter aims to give you the confidence to choose an appropriate and top-quality supplement for your dog, whatever his age or ailment.

DOES YOUR DOG NEED A SUPPLEMENT?

Healthy dogs should not, in theory, require any supplements. However, we live in a less than perfect world. In reality, our dogs are not always getting a diet of a wide range of freshly prepared, 100 per cent organic meat, colourful vegetables and fruits, in a completely stress-free environment. Commonly, the nutritional value of food is lost through intensive farming, processing and cooking. This is especially the case for dogs fed on commercially prepared, mass-produced foods such as cans or biscuits. Added to this, remember that manufacturers attempt to balance the nutrients in their diets based on guidelines for an average dog. But as each dog is an individual and will differ in how well they digest and utilize their food, not all of them will thrive on these diets. This is how the need for supplements arises. Another situation where the use of supplements is usually warranted is if your dog is unwell, and hence has an increased need for particular building blocks to help his body repair and heal. Older dogs too are prime candidates for dietary supplements, to help support the degenerative changes relating to old age.

HOW TO CHOOSE A SUPPLEMENT

While veterinary medicines are under the jurisdiction of the Veterinary Medicines Directorate (VMD), supplements are classed as complementary feedstuffs and are regulated, somewhat less stringently, by the European Food Safety Authority (EFSA) and local authority Trading Standards. Studies have shown that some nutraceuticals are mislabelled, contain impurities, and can contain variable

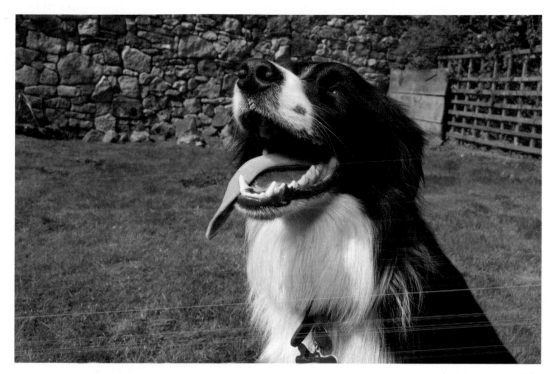

Supplements can help to maintain health.

quantities of active ingredients. With so many different supplements now available, and the huge variation between them in terms of quality, cost and effectiveness, you can (and should) be fussy. Don't be put off though, as there are some really excellent, top-quality supplements out there (often even better than human products) that will be of enormous benefit to your dog. It's just that you may have to do your homework, and a little comparing, before you find them. Don't be afraid to contact the manufacturers directly if you need more information on their product. The following are the key guidelines for helping you select high-quality supplements. Focus on purity, quality and quantity and you won't go far wrong.

How much active ingredient does it contain and what is its purity? This can vary widely, from high human-grade ingredients to those with hardly any active constituent in them at all. Also appreciate that the active component needs to be in a form that your dog can utilize, in order to be effective (see Bioavailability below).

What other ingredients does it contain? All ingredients should be listed on the label. If you are unsure, ask the manufacturer what the purpose of each ingredient is and why it is included.

Where is it sourced? Find out where the product comes from and how it is manufactured, so that you can be sure that it is ethically and sustainably produced. This is especially important for supplements such as chondroitin, which can potentially come from shark cartilage; with any fish supplement, make sure it's not from wild-caught stock.

Will using an equivalent human supplement be just as good? For example, if both of you take glucosamine for your achy joints, or an antioxidant to support your immune system, can you give your supplement to your dog? The answer is, 'It depends'. In some instances both of your supplements will be identical except that his has a picture of a dog on the label. However, in most cases your dog's supplement will have been specifically formulated to be more effective and palatable for him. Always pay attention to the quality and quantity of the active ingredient, and buy the best and most appropriate one for your dog.

What is the dose and what is the cost per day? Do check this, because it can be misleading. Work out how much of the supplement your dog will need per day, and hence what it will cost on a daily basis. This will allow you to compare prices. Cheaper compounds are less likely to offer high quality; you usually do get what you pay for.

What formulation is it and will your dog take it? Only you know how fussy your dog can be. Sometimes it is easier to get a liquid formulation if it is difficult to give your dog tablets. Read the small print and see whether the supplement needs to go with food or if it should be given directly into his mouth.

Check it has a batch number and expiry date This is a legal requirement.

What are the health claims and is there any data or research to back these up? Supplements are not allowed to make any specific claims that they can be used to 'treat', let alone 'cure', a named condition. There are strict guidelines that only allow them to use broad phrases such as 'promote' or 'improve' health.

Make yourself aware of any potential side effects Usually supplements are relatively safe to use. However, there can be side effects, and supplements can contain contaminants that will also cause problems. This is why the use of any supplements needs to be under the guidance of your vet.

Instructions for use The label should give recommendations for daily amounts, including information on how the supplement needs to be stored.

Scientific evidence Some companies have begun providing data for their products through independent scientific studies (but be aware that testimonials are not the same as evidence of proof, they are simply someone's opinion).

GENERAL GUIDELINES FOR USE OF SUPPLEMENTS

Firstly, be aware that supplements work slowly and it is likely to take several weeks before you start to notice any benefits. It is also a good idea to introduce them slowly; start by giving your dog half the recommended dose for a few weeks, before building up to the full amount. This enables his body to get used to it, and in the rare instances where there are any sensitivities, these can be addressed. The exception to this is glucosamine supplements. These are

The efficacy of herbal supplements can vary, depending on the method of harvest and manufacture as well as the species of plant used.

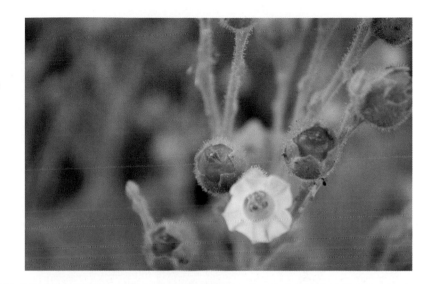

WHAT'S NOT ON THE LABEL

Unlike medicines, which are strictly regulated and controlled, supplements are not currently subject to such rigorous quality controls. This can leave you in a vulnerable position when you are picking a supplement off the shelf for your dog. The manufacturer needs to list every ingredient in the supplement. They must also state the amount of any ingredient that they have drawn attention to, such as 'herbal coat conditioning tablets with ginger'. In this case the label should state the amount of ginger it contains. However, even when the amount of the active ingredient is given, spot-checking to verify the claim is not common. In addition, remember that supplements are not allowed to make any specific claims that they can be used to 'treat' a 'named condition'. They have to use broad phrases and general statements. Happily, all this is set to change, with tighter regulations for supplements due in the near future.

usually given at a double dose to begin with, and then reduced down to a maintenance level after a number of weeks.

Remember that supplements need to be used appropriately and carefully and are never a substitute for a good diet or normal veterinary care. Do check with your vet before you start your dog on a supplement, to make sure that it is suitable for him. Also let your vet know if he has a reaction to any supplement.

Bioavailability

Bioavailability is a measure of how effectively a supplement can be used by the body. For instance, it may be the highest quality, most expensive supplement, but if it is parcelled up into a capsule, or chemically bonded to another constituent that makes it difficult for the body to use, then it is effectively useless. High bioavailability means that the active constituent of the supplement will be

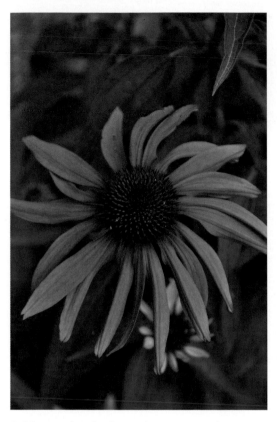

Echinacea is a herb used to support the immune system.

highly reactive molecules that are made in the body all the time; they are a natural waste product of many everyday processes. However, stress and exposure to toxins in food and the environment cause an increased production. Free radicals damage cells and are involved in many chronic, degenerative conditions. Antioxidants are the body's natural defence against free radicals and are provided, in part, by the array of fresh foods in the diet. They play a key role in maintaining health and preventing disease. The following list of antioxidants will be found in colourful, sun-ripened fruit and vegetables, as well as in meat. You don't need to worry too much about the names on the list; they are just there so that you can recognize them when you see them on the label of an antioxidant supplement.

What are they used for?
Most dogs will be exposed to the factors that cause increased free-radical production on a daily basis, from the pollution in the air that they breathe to the pesticide

able to be used to maximum effect by your dog. Of course bioavailability is something that the manufacturer of the supplement should be aware of, but it is still a factor that you should check when selecting a supplement.

A ROUGH GUIDE TO THE MOST COMMONLY USED SUPPLEMENTS

Antioxidants
What are they and what do they do?
Antioxidants are substances that help to protect the body from the damaging effects of free radicals. Free radicals are

---

LIST OF COMMON ANTIOXIDANTS

Vitamin C (ascorbic acid)
Vitamin E (tocopherols)
Alpha-lipoic acid (ALA)
Beta carotene
Bioflavinoids
Coenzyme Q10
Grape seed extract
Green tea extract
Milk thistle
SAM-e
Selenium
Superoxide dismutase

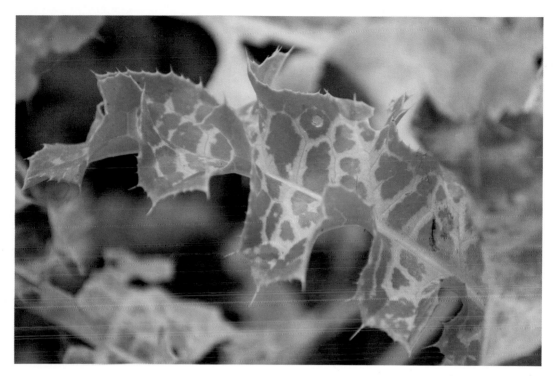

Milk thistle is an important antioxidant.

residues in the foods that they eat. Therefore, antioxidants will be a valuable supplement for a lot of dogs. However, they may be particularly beneficial for elderly dogs and those suffering from degenerative conditions. They can also play a role in supporting dogs suffering from immune mediated diseases, as well as cancer. Antioxidants help to promote recovery after serious illness, and are often given to dogs that are on ongoing medications.

Essential fatty acids
What are they and what do they do?
Essential fatty acids (EFAs) are essential components of your dog's daily diet. They are crucial to every cell in his body, and aid in the regulation of nearly every bodily function. They play a key role in helping to regulate the immune system, and can act as powerful anti-inflammatories. EFAs are also particularly important for maintaining a healthy skin and coat, for brain and kidney function and for a healthy heart. The most important families of fatty acids are the omega-3s and the omega-6s. Most plant oils contain both types but in different ratios, so are better suited for certain conditions than others.

The omega-3s, Eicosapentaenoic acid (EPA) and Docosahexaenoic acid (DHA), are principally found in fish oils. Rich sources are the deep sea, cold-water fish such as salmon, mackerel, halibut and herring. Flax seed oil is one of the richest plant sources of the omega-3 oil Alpha-linolenic acid (ALA). The omega-6s, Gamma Linolenic acid (GLA) and Linoleic acid (LA), are readily derived from most vegetable and plant oils, as well as some meat and dairy products. Borage is a very good source of omega-6, much more concentrated than Evening Primrose oil. Not only is it important to have enough of these oils, it is also crucial to have the right balance. This is because the ratio of omega-3 to omega-6 influences whether they promote or reduce inflammation, and hence will differ depending on every dog's individual requirements. Often the easiest way of achieving a good balance is to use one of the many proprietary EFA supplements that are now readily available. These should also contain a source of vitamin E (Tocopherol), which must always be added when supplementing with EFAs. To ensure that you choose a supplement of the best quality, look for one that is made by cold pressing. Try and buy your EFA supplement in small quanti-ties for freshness and stability, because after opening it will only remain opti-mally effective for up to three months. Regarding fish-oil supplements, choose ones that were sustainably fished, and also pay particular attention to the manufacturing process. The time bet-ween the salmon being fished and having its oils extracted needs to be as short as possible. Salmon oil is usually considered the gold standard, as it can be farmed in fresh water and so has less risk of heavy metal contamination.

What are they used for?

A balanced omega supplement can be used to help maintain overall health in most dogs. Otherwise choose a supple-ment that is specifically rich in omega-3 for dogs with heart conditions and those with kidney disease. Omega-3 is also used to support the immune system and to help promote healthy brain function in ageing dogs, as well as for healthy joints.

OMEGA-3 AND OMEGA-6 SOURCES

Using EFA supplements is all about balance. While omega-3s can be used on their own for conditions such as heart or brain function, when the omega-6s are called for they are best used in combination with an omega-3. The richest sources of omega-3s are fish, namely cold-water, oily fish such as salmon, herring, mackerel, anchovies and sardines. These are all full of Docosahexaenoic acid (DHA) and Eicosapentaenoic acid (EPA), which are the chemical names for the omega-3s. Green-lipped Mussel (Perna Canaliculus) is another rich source of omega-3. There is also a type of omega-3 called Alpha-linolenic acid (ALA) which is found in plants, most importantly in flax seed oil (and also in walnuts and hemp seed oil). However, in order for it to play its role in the conditions that specifically call for omega-3 supplementation, such as heart, brain, eye or joint health, ALA needs to have been first converted to EPA. Hence for these conditions it would be better to use an omega-3 from fish oils. But in most cases of maintenance of overall skin and coat health, ALA is ideal and does not need any conversion. Finally, although commonly given, cod liver oil is not a beneficial supplement for your dog. This is because it contains high levels of vitamins A and D, which if given daily can build up and cause toxicity.

Feeding oily fish once a week can be another excellent, but less concentrated, way of providing omega-3s. However, avoid using tinned fish as the tinning process destroys most of the useful omega-3. A balanced omega-3/omega-6 supplement is often recommended for promoting a healthy skin and coat. Look for supplements that include ALA, LA and GLA. They are used for dogs that suffer from skin allergies as they can help to reduce itching and improve dry, flaky skin.

Glucosamine and related products
What are they and what do they do?
Glucosamines are complex sugar-type molecules that are produced naturally in the body. They are used for the repair of connective tissues, such as cartilage, by stimulating the production of glyco-saminoglycans (GAGs). Glucosamines can be refined from natural sources, usually from shellfish, and given as supplements to augment the body's own production. This is especially necessary when demand exceeds the body's normal production, such as in old age and arthritis. There is significant evidence to support their efficacy, and they are widely used in the management of degenerative joint disease. However, these supplements do much more than help repair and rebuild cartilage, they actually act to slow down its destruction. In addition, glucosamine has also been shown to have anti-inflammatory activity, helping to relieve some of the joint pain in arthritis. It can be in

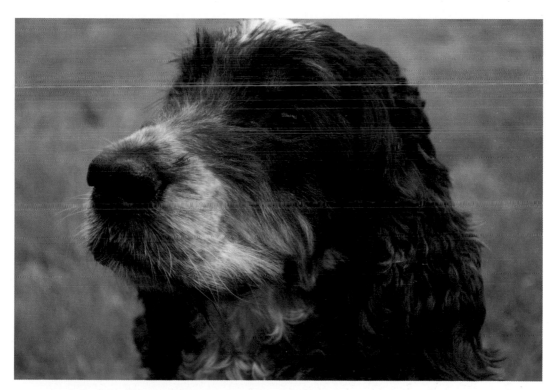

Essential fatty acids help to promote a healthy skin and coat.

one of two forms in the supplement, as a hydrochloride (HCl) or as a sulphate. It is widely agreed that the glucosamine HCl formulation is the higher-quality, purer form, and hence more effective. As well as being used on its own, glucosamine is commonly combined with other active constituents such as chondroitin sulfate. This is a related compound (usually derived from bovine or poultry sources, or from shellfish) that works by helping to reduce cartilage destruction. In addition methylsulfonylmethane (MSM) is often combined with the glucosamine and chondroitin for suggested further benefits. The Green-lipped Mussel (*Perna canaliculus*) is cultivated exclusively in the pure coastal waters around New Zealand and is an excellent and unique natural source of glucosamine and chondroitin. It also contains Eicosatetraenoic acids (ETAs), which are a special type of omega-3 fatty acids that provide it with additional anti-inflammatory effects.

Be sure to source your glucosamine supplement carefully so that it contains adequate amounts of active ingredients for it to be effective. The maintenance level for a medium-sized dog is around 500mg glucosamine daily. It is also important that the supplement is ethically sourced and that the chondroitin does not come from shark cartilage, for example. Be wary of non-specific categorization such as 'marine sources'. There are vegetarian forms of this supplement available that use a grain source of chondroitin and derive their glucosamine from microorganisms.

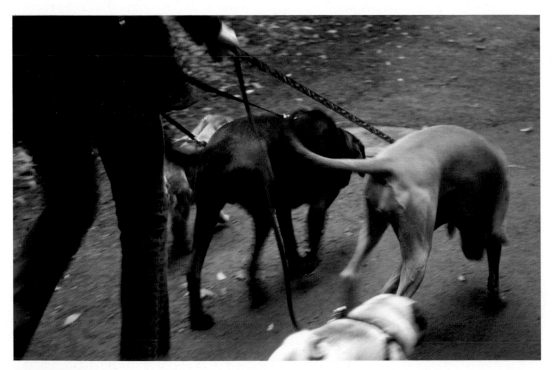

Glucosamines help with mobility.

What are they used for?

The body has an increased requirement for glucosamines in ageing, disease and after injury. Glucosamine is therefore a highly valuable supplement for conditions such as arthritis, degenerative joint disease (including those affecting the spine), hip dysplasia, and in ligament and tendon injuries. These supplements have maximum benefit if they are used as early as possible in the onset of the condition. They are usually given at a higher dosage for an initial period of several weeks, after which they are given at an ongoing maintenance level every day.

Probiotics

What are they and what do they do?

Your dog's digestive system is home to millions of beneficial bacteria that help him to process his food, ward off harmful bacteria and support his immune system. They are also a good source of B vitamins. Many factors can harm and alter the gut flora, including stress, anxiety, upset tummies, as well as antibiotics and other medications. This can have serious knock-on effects for your dog's immune system as well as his digestion, as it gives the harmful bacteria a chance to proliferate. As a result he may suffer from symptoms such as constipation or loose stools, bloating, flatulence and possible food sensitivities. Probiotics are supplements that contain healthy bacteria, usually several strains such as Acidophilus, Lactobacillus, Bifodobacterium, among others. They act to restore and rebalance the population of microorganisms in the gut and so strengthen the immune system. Most probiotic supplements will also contain a source of prebiotics. These are the fermentable fibres such as fructo-oligosaccharides (FOS) that feed the good bacteria and help them to provide a more

lasting effect. Contrary to popular opinion a daily serving of live yoghurt isn't sufficient. High-quality products, usually available as either powder or capsules, are much better as they are far more concentrated and are especially formulated to protect the bacteria from your dog's stomach acid. Each capsule or teaspoon of probiotic will contain literally millions of bacteria specific to the canine digestive system, helping to repopulate and restore the correct

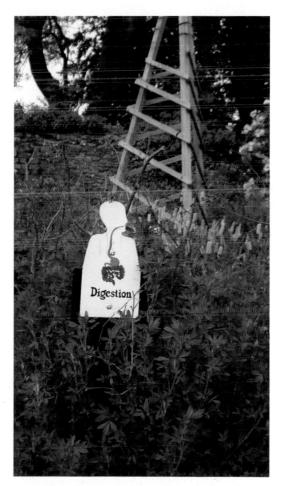

Probiotics and herbal remedies can aid digestive complaints.

balance. Using a probiotic supplement that is specific for dogs (as opposed to one for humans) will have the benefit of providing canine-specific bacteria that will be 'alive and kicking' when they reach the dog's intestinal tract. Probiotics may need to be kept in the fridge to keep them viable.

What are they used for?
Any form of digestive upset, such as diarrhoea, constipation, bloating or dietary sensitivities or after treatment of a heavy worm burden. In addition, probiotics are often given as a follow-up to a prolonged course of antibiotics (as these can affect the good bacteria as well as destroying the harmful ones). They can also be used proactively at times when you can predict your dog will be under stress, such as going to kennels, moving house or even just having a change in diet (all occasions that can upset the normal balance of his intestinal flora). They can also be used routinely in old age and in convalescence.

Vitamins and minerals
What are they and what do they do?
Vitamins are chemical compounds that are essential for your dog's everyday body processes, in other words his metabolism. They are required in tiny amounts for all the chemical reactions that go on all the time to keep him alive.

Some vitamins are actually a group of related compounds that have the same function. Each vitamin is typically used in many different reactions and consequently usually has many roles in the body. Fat-soluble vitamins A, D, E and K are absorbed from the gut along with fat and can be stored in the body, so a daily intake is not required. However, if too much is stored, toxicity can occur, which is why the dosage of vitamin supplements must be carefully controlled. Conversely, the water-soluble vitamins C and B complex cannot be stored in the body in significant amounts and a daily intake is required. The best source of vitamins for your dog is fresh, wholesome food. One interesting difference between dogs and humans is that dogs can make their own vitamin C. However, this doesn't mean that it isn't an important supplement under certain conditions, such as during stress or disease when your dog's production is likely to be reduced (see the table on page 120 for a list of important vitamins for your dog).

Minerals are essential for the correct growth, development and everyday life processes of your dog. There are eighteen minerals that are important for your dog; some are called macrominerals as they are required in larger amounts, while others are called trace elements. Macrominerals such as calcium and phosphorus make up bone tissue. Trace minerals, such as zinc and selenium, are needed in tiny amounts but play key roles in how your dog's body works. The amount of each mineral must be in balance in the body. This is because they all interact with each other. Too much of one can interfere with the absorption or availability of another. With such complex interactions and potential knock-on effects, when using anything other than broad-spectrum multivitamin or mineral supplements, veterinary guidance is important.

What are they used for?
A well-formulated multivitamin and mineral supplement is likely to be beneficial to most dogs. However, it is potentially dangerous to supplement with a

single vitamin or mineral. If a high dose of a specific mineral or vitamin is required (to rectify a deficiency for example) then it will be important to use it under the guidance of your vet. This way you will be sure to maintain a proper balance.

LESS COMMONLY USED SUPPLEMENTS

Alfalfa Alfalfa is a member of the pea family, is considered highly nourishing, and is a rich source of many trace minerals. It is also a rich source of protein and dietary fibre, and vitamins A, B complex, C, D, E and K. Alfalfa also contains chlorophyll, which acts as an antioxidant.

Bioflavinoids These are plant pigments giving colour to many fruits and vegetables, and are especially rich in most berries. Bioflavinoids are usually good sources of vitamin C and are often described as nature's 'cure all'. They have wide-ranging effects, including anti-allergy, anti-inflammatory, antiviral and anti-cancer properties, as well as being powerful antioxidants.

Bee Propolis Propolis is a resin-like material used by bees; it acts like the immune system of the hive. It is considered an excellent antibacterial substance and may also enhance the immune system. (Caution: some dogs can be allergic to bee products.)

L-carnitine This is a vitamin-like compound that is essential for converting fat into energy. It is present naturally in meat and dairy products, and is added to most commercial diets. Supplementation may be beneficial in many conditions, including heart disease, lethargy and poor physical stamina. (Note that L-carnitine is the preferred form over D-carnitine.)

Coenzyme Q10 Also known as ubiquinone, this is an enzyme that plays a vital role in energy production in the body. It is present in most foods but can be lost through cooking and preparation. It is thought to be especially beneficial for elderly dogs, for whom it may help to support the age-related decline in immunity. It also has a specific role in periodontal and gum disease.

Dimethylglycine (DMG) This is a vitamin-like substance found naturally in meat, seeds and grains. It may enhance metabolism and is used to support the immune system and aid recovery.

Garlic This herb has a very long history of powerful medicinal effects. It contains the active constituent allicin, and is also a rich source of fatty acids, B and C vitamins and selenium. It could be renamed 'nature's own antibiotic and antiseptic'. It also has antiviral effects and is a powerful support for the immune system. Use of a small amount in your dog's diet occasionally is beneficial. However, large amounts of garlic given regularly over extended periods have the potential to cause toxicity, so should not be used.

Grape seed extract This contains a very special type of bioflavinoid called a proanthocyanidin, which is more powerful than many others. It is often used for dogs following strokes, brain damage or seizures. However, do be aware that whole grapes are poisonous to dogs and therefore should not be given to them.

Glutamine Glutamine is an important energy source for cells of the digestive tract. Whenever the digestive tract is stressed, the need for glutamine is increased. This makes it of benefit in cases of inflammatory bowel disease, as well as in diarrhoea. Natural sources include pearl barley, wheat bran and oats.

Kelp and other seaweed supplements Kelp is the most common seaweed supplement. Seaweed can be a rich source of minerals, vitamins and trace elements, particularly iodine. Iodine is necessary for the correct functioning of the thyroid gland (which regulates your dog's metabolic rate). It should be used under veterinary supervision only in dogs with thyroid disease.

Milk thistle This is the favourite herbal liver protector. Milk thistle's active ingredient, silymarin, works as a powerful antioxidant and has also been shown to help regenerate and repair injured liver cells. Hence it is especially beneficial for dogs with liver disease or damage, as well as those on daily medications that are metabolized in the liver.

SAM-e (S-adenosylemethionine) This is a natural biochemical product made in the body by the amino acid methionine. It is used as a liver support supplement.

USING SUPPLEMENTS FOR POSITIVE HEALTH

To summarize, the best way of using some of the supplements outlined in this chapter is to prevent your dog getting ill. For example, now you know that by giving him a probiotic supplement at times when he may be under stress, you can help to ward off the potential for a tummy upset. Equally, now that you are aware of how glucosamines work, you can speak to your vet about using them at the very earliest signs of your dog stiffening up with arthritis. You have also learnt how borage oil, as a great source of omega-6s, can help the dog with the scurfy coat, while fish oils have a role for the ageing brain. The list goes on, but you can see how supplements can be used to great effect to promote 'positive health'. One of the most important factors in using any supplement is their role in helping the body's own self-regulatory mechanisms repair and maintain healthy function. Remember, the wrong balance of supplements, or over-supplementation, can be harmful, so always use them appropriately.

Your vet may suggest a supplement for your dog.

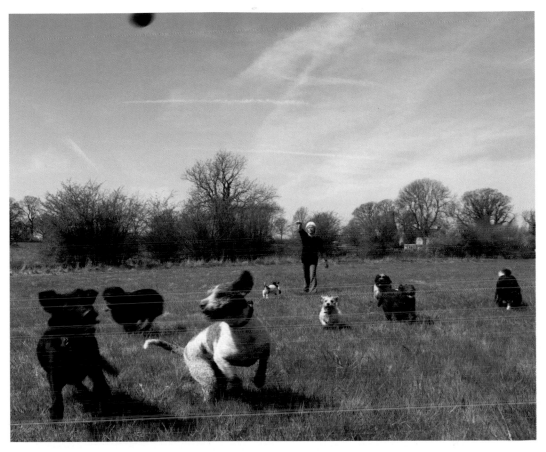

Use supplements to help maintain your dog's flexibility and mobility.

LIST OF CONDITIONS AND SUGGESTED SUPPLEMENTS

Skin and coat Omega-6/omega-3s.

Immune Support (for cancer, immunodeficiency diseases, chronic diseases) Antioxidants, vitamin C.

Cardiovascular Support Omega-3s.

Joint/Musculoskeletal Glucosamine and chondroitin, green-lipped mussel.

Liver support Milk thistle, SAM-e, multivitamins and minerals.

Ageing Antioxidants, multivitamins and minerals.

Allergies Antioxidants, omega-3s.

Neurological Antioxidants (especially grape seed extract), omega-3s.

Important vitamins for your dog

Vitamin	Common/other name of vitamin	Common sources	What it is used for	Comments
A	Retinol	Liver, fish oils, eggs and dairy products.	Normal growth, development and reproduction. For good eyesight.	Beware that vitamin is stored in the liver and excess supplementation could lead to toxicity (why cod liver oil is not recommended).
D	D_2 ergocalciferol, D_3 cholecalciferol	Synthesis by sunlight's UV radiation in the skin. Or preformed in the diet from fish oils, egg yolks and dairy products.	Important in skeletal development and tooth production.	
E	Tocopherol (natural forms have a prefix d-, while synthetic forms have a prefix dl-).	Vegetable oils, seeds, grains, bran and wheat-germ.	An important antioxidant – protects EFAs from damage.	Need to supplement vitamin E if you are using an EFA supplement. (Usually contained already in proprietary EFA supplements.)
K		Intestinal bacteria. Leafy greens, alfalfa, seeds, liver and fish.	For blood clotting.	
B	Thiamin (B_1), Riboflavin (B_2), Niacin (B_3), Pantothenic acid (B_5), Pyridoxine (B_6), Folic acid, Biotin, B_{12} (and Choline).	The dog's intestinal flora, whole grains, brewer's yeast, liver, beans, dairy products, nuts, green vegetables.	Essential for energy production, growth and for a healthy immune system.	Vegetarian diets may need supplementation. If intestinal flora has been reduced then supplements may be needed.
C	Ascorbic acid or sodium ascorbate.	Fruits (especially citrus), vegetables and organ meats.	Primary function is the production of collagen, the main protein substance in the body. Important for wound repair and healthy gums. A crucial antioxidant, vital for the immune system.	Dogs produce their own vitamin C. However, stress and illness increases requirements far above this, so supplements are commonly beneficial.

8 THE ELDERLY DOG

Old age is not a disease; it is just a natural slowing down. In many ways looking after your dog in his twilight years will be similar to how you treated him as a puppy. The cycle of life seems to go full circle as the old dog reverts back to puppyhood in his behaviour and needs. There is no denying that elderly dogs can be slow and grumpy, not to mention smelly. However, after a lifetime of companionship, showing your elderly dog patience and a few extra moments to catch up on a walk is a small price to pay. The more you know about the ageing process, the better prepared you'll be for the changes that you may notice in your dog. By appreciating the physical as well as the emotional and mental changes that occur in the ageing body, you will have more tolerance for his slowness and eccentricities. This chapter will cover the important issues that relate to old age in dogs, from how to cope with incontinence and senility to the various treatment options for arthritis. By helping you to see the world from your elderly friend's point of view, you will start to spot ways to help him navigate his way through his daily life more easily. It will become clear that by simply making a few small changes to his everyday care – his bed, diet, and exercise routine, for example – you can make a great difference to your elderly dog's comfort and health. We will also discover how natural, holistic therapies are especially suited to the elderly dog. They treat the mind and body as one and can help to improve the more subtle signs of ageing such as depression, confusion and insomnia. Remember the wisdom of the elderly dog, treat him with respect and patience and savour each day in his company.

THE AGEING PROCESS

Our domestic dog's wild forebear, the wolf, does not experience old age. Mother nature is harsh; these animals die of exposure, starvation and disease at between five and seven years old. They just wouldn't survive if they suffered from arthritis, let alone senility. Our dogs, on

---

DOG YEARS

We used to equate one year of a dog's life to seven human years. This was based on the life expectancy of ten years for dogs and seventy for people. Clearly this is now different as both of us are living longer. A more accurate comparison may now be nearer to one dog year to five and a half human years. We tend to classify large-breed dogs as senior at around five years, and small dogs, who live longer, are regarded as elderly when they are about seven or eight.

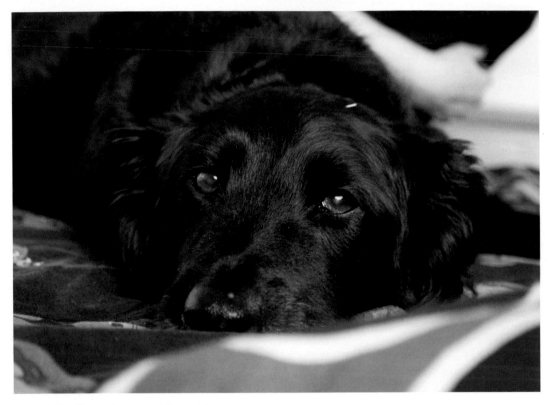

An elderly dog relaxing while she has acupuncture.

the other hand, have a much more comfortable lifestyle and can live long into their teens. There is some debate as to the age of the world's oldest dog. It seems that the Dachshund from Shrewsbury that reached twenty had already been pipped at the post a long time before by Bluey, an Australian cattle dog who died aged twenty-nine in 1939. The question is: when does a dog become 'senior' or 'geriatric'? There is not a standard answer; it will be different for every individual. As a general rule large and giant-breed dogs have a shorter lifespan, around eight to ten years, and show signs of ageing earlier, while small and medium-sized dogs can live to around fifteen to sixteen years old. This puts paid to the well-known idea of one human year being equivalent to seven 'dog' years. The relationship is not linear, because of the variation in life spans and rates of ageing between dogs and humans. A more accurate, up-to-date comparison may be that of around five and a half human years being the equivalent of one 'dog' year. Research has shown that the most important factors that determine your dog's lifespan, apart from his genes, are his diet, his activity level, and any previous or ongoing medical problems.

SIGNS OF OLD AGE

The signs of ageing will be more or less the same for every dog. These include a greying around the muzzle, creaky joints, a slowing-up on walks, and some stiffness on first getting up in the mornings. In addition, deterioration in eyesight and hearing may make your dog less responsive and interactive with you. He may also appear forgetful and confused. Some signs of ageing are, however, less obvious from the outside. These relate to deterioration in the functioning of your dog's internal organs, namely his liver, kidneys and heart, after a lifetime's filtering, detoxifying and pumping of blood. This is why any noticeable alterations in an older dog's drinking habits, appetite or indeed general demeanour, as well as the more obvious stiff joints and reduced mobility, should be an indication to have him checked by the vet. Never assume that any change in your elderly dog's behaviour or physical condition is simply due to old age, because the signs of ageing and those of several medical conditions will be indistinguishable to the untrained eye. Thus, regular medical checks for your elderly dog are more important than they were in his early years. This means that any problems can be picked up and treated at an early stage. Finally, by turning to Ancient Chinese medicine we can begin to understand how the signs of ageing in mind and body are part of a whole, explained by a lack of kidney qi. According to the philosophy of Traditional Chinese Medicine, kidney qi is lost throughout life, so old animals necessarily have less of it. This energy is associated with the bones, the hair on the head, the sense of hearing, and the emotion of fear. So we can see how this is linked to arthritis, greying of the muzzle, deafness and the fear and anxiety of old age.

Now dogs are living longer than ever before, understanding the ageing process and knowing how to care for the geriatric dog is becoming more important. Turning to ancient wisdom seems an appropriate way of understanding it.

CARING FOR YOUR ELDERLY DOG

There is a fine line between easing your dog's transition into old age, where he may need to take things steadier, and ushering him into the life of a canine invalid. Where sensible, and if he seems healthy and comfortable, it is best to let him set his own limits as to what he still wants to do. This means that instead of assuming that he will still be fine on a nine-mile hike at age ten, you go on a four-mile walk and let him explore as far as he wants off the lead, to make up any extra exercise he wants. Some dogs are troubled very little by signs of ageing, while for others aches, pains, incontinence or senility can make their everyday life uncomfortable or distressing. So while we don't need to install handrails or Stannah stairlifts, there are a few easy ways to make your dog's home environment more comfortable for him. These are outlined below.

Mobility

Reduced mobility is likely to be the most obvious issue for most elderly dogs, as they start to seize up with arthritis. Your dog may have trouble going up and down steps and getting into and out of the car. In larger dogs, a stiff neck may make it uncomfortable to reach down to his food or water bowl. To ease these problems and help make life easier for him, use of steps and stair gates, ramps and raised food bowls can be considered. Be inventive, you don't need to buy expensive equipment: adapt a crate as a step, or use a cushion to help him get up onto his favourite chair. If your elderly dog is weak, wobbly or prone to sliding around on wooden, laminate or polished floors, then laying down carpets or rugs will make a huge difference to his quality of life.

Comfort and warmth

Attention to what sort of bed your ageing dog sleeps on is important. Consider using an orthopaedic bed, which is firmer and moulds to support his tender joints and provide extra comfort. Equally, consider how easy it is for your dog to get into and out of his bed. Ensuring the sides are not too high, and that it is not in a position that makes it awkward for him to get into it, will be helpful. If he is a dog that prefers to stretch out on the floor, rather than in a bed, provide him with a blanket or pad. Older dogs are usually more sensitive to the cold and benefit from a soft, warm bed away from draughts. For those that really do suffer from the cold, heated pads or good old-fashioned woolly blankets are a necessary addition in the winter. The elderly dog may also benefit from a coat when you take him out on chilly winter walks, as old bones definitely feel the cold more than young ones (lack of kidney yang).

Daily care

Your elderly dog may need some help with his daily ablutions, as eyes can become dry and ears crusty in old age. Wipe away any sleep or discharge from his eyes every morning, using warm water on cotton wool, and use Euphrasia drops if they seem red (*see* Chapter 9). Brushing your dog's teeth is another important daily task. The same goes for a daily grooming, which, as well as acting like a massage, allows you to give his body a good once-over to check for any lumps or masses that can occur with age. A quick rub to his legs and feet every morning when he first gets up can help to get your dog's circulation going, easing arthritic pains and helping to prevent stumbling. Finally, more regular nail clipping (including the dew claws) is usually another part of routine elderly dog care, as he will be wearing his nails down less on walks.

Incontinence

The involuntary leaking of urine during sleep can be one of the trials of old age, especially in bitches. It can be a complex condition, linked to causes that range from confusion and senility to physical deterioration of the urinary tract, such as weakening of the valve that holds urine in the bladder. Your vet will be able to identify the cause and suggest the most appropriate treatment for your dog. As well as addressing any specific causal factors for the incontinence, you can make a significant difference by just ensuring that your elderly dog gets plenty of opportunities to go outside and empty his bladder. This prevents him having to hold on and put increased pressure on his weakened bladder muscles. In fact, for very elderly, senile dogs, you may need to remember for them and take them outside every so often (even if this means waking them up) to ensure that they go to the toilet. If they don't make it out in time, having floors that are easily cleaned and dog bedding that is absorbent and draws the leakage away from his body are obviously a great help. Complementary treatments such as acupuncture and homeopathy are gentle and can be effective methods of treating urinary incontinence, with no side effects.

*Holistic treatment for
urinary incontinence*
Acupuncture works by raising the body's yang energy and stimulating neurological function to strengthen bladder control. Homeopathic remedies such as Causticum and Sepia are two of the most commonly indicated remedies for the unconscious leaking of urine during sleep. Herbs that strengthen the urinary tract include dandelion leaf, nettle, cleavers and parsley. Using the leaves of these plants as an infusion, added to your dog's food, can help maintain bladder tone (*see* Chapter 1).

Losing control of bowel function, although less common, is unfortunately much more problematic and difficult to treat either by conventional or complementary means. Living with and managing an elderly dog that can no longer control his bowels is not pleasant for either of you. As well as the obvious hygiene concerns of faecal incontinence, there is the distress that it evidently causes your dog. Apart from ruling out a tummy upset and loose stools or diarrhoea playing a part, this is generally not a condition that can be successfully treated. In fact It Is often one of the issues to take into account when you are weighing up the various aspects that affect your dog's quality of life, and whether it is fair to keep him going when life is far from dignified for him.

Sleep patterns and yin deficiency
Changes to the sleep/wake cycle are another sign of ageing. Old animals tend to have plenty of short naps during the day and to sleep less at night. This change of behaviour can be explained by the Traditional Chinese Medicine concept of the opposite but equal qualities of yin and yang. Yang is the active, daytime energy, and yin is the restful, quiet energy of the night. In young healthy dogs these yin and yang energies are exactly balanced by the day and night of the twenty-four-hour cycle. However, in aged dogs there is less of the restful yin energy that should predominate at night, as it has been used up during their lifetime. This means that a relative excess of the active yang energy troubles them at night, making them seem hot and restless. Acupuncture treatment to rebalance their yin and yang energies can therefore be helpful for those dogs that suffer night-time restlessness and insomnia.

There are of course other reasons that may be causing your dog to be restless at night, barking, whining or pacing in the small hours. He may be in pain, finding it difficult to lie down comfortably due to arthritis, or confused and anxious due to senile changes in his behaviour. Equally, it may be due to his weak bladder and heightened thirst making him need to go to the toilet more often at night, or changes in his appetite patterns making him feel hungry at odd times. This is why having your dog checked over by the vet if he can't settle at night will help you identify the cause and treat any underlying medical issues. Another reason for night-time restlessness is linked to brain ageing, or to deteriorating eyesight and hearing making your dog feel more vulnerable in the dark and when he is on his own (see Anxiety, below). In this instance, allowing him to sleep nearer to you, or leaving a dim light and a radio on low may prove soothing and reassuring.

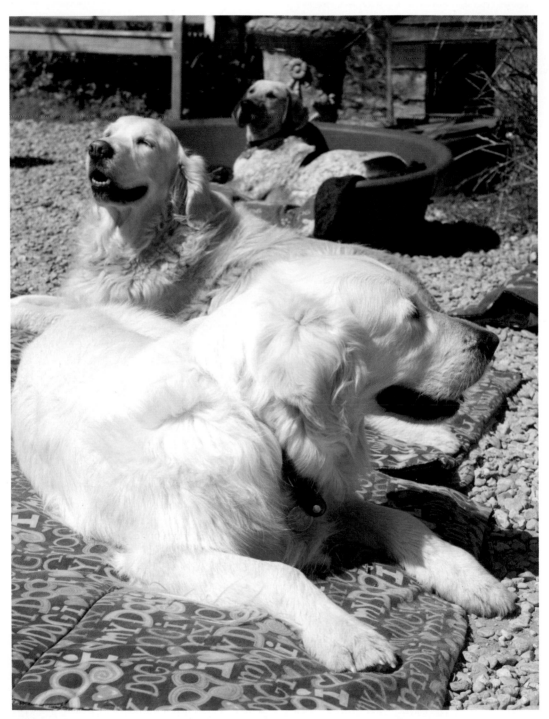

These old friends are enjoying a snooze in the sun.

*Holistic treatment for
sleep disturbances*

Adding four drops of Dr Bach's Rescue Remedy to your dog's evening meal, or onto a treat before bed, may help him to settle and rest during the night. Using herbal remedies such as valerian (often combined with skullcap) as an aid to better sleep is also well documented in dogs. It has a gentle sedative effect, calming the nerves and relaxing the body ready for sleep. Finally, one or two drops of lavender oil on a cushion or blanket near your dog's bed may help soothe and calm him and enhance his sleep patterns (avoid using it directly on his bed in case he is sensitive to it).

In summary

Caring for your dog as he grows old is simply a question of trying to put yourself in his shoes to see which parts of his daily life he seems to struggle with and what practical steps you can take to make life easier for him. Be inventive, and don't forget that even if you make just one small change, this can have a big impact on his quality of life over weeks and months.

HOW TO IMPROVE LIFE FOR YOUR ELDERLY DOG

Daily one-to-one time

Daily massage and grooming

Special walks on his own, little and often

Ensure his bed supports arthritic joints

A quiet place to sleep

More toilet trips

Senior diet – little and often feeding, and watch for obesity.

DETERIORATING SENSES

Deterioration in hearing and eyesight are inevitable parts of the ageing process. This altered perception and awareness of the world around him may, if significant, affect how your dog behaves and interacts with you. For example, if he can't hear you coming towards him or even recognize you from a distance, then he may well startle as you approach. If he is frightened or taken off guard like this, your dog could even snap or seem aggressive because he is frightened. This uncharacteristic behaviour may be seen in his responses towards other dogs too, because if your dog can't see or hear them properly, then he will not be able to read their signals and work out whether they are friend or foe. Having said that, you will often find that other dogs do seem to pick up on the fact that elderly dogs are more fragile, and well-socialized dogs will usually be gentle and respectful towards a senior dog.

Eyesight

As he ages, your dog's eyes will become cloudy due to changes in the lens. Like us as we age, our dog's near vision diminishes more quickly than his distant vision. This explains why he can still pick out silhouettes on the horizon when on a walk, but may bump into chair and table legs at home. If your dog is losing his sight, make navigating his way around at home easier for him by keeping furniture in the same place and providing plenty of room for him to manoeuvre between his usual spots. Help guide him on walks by using positive, definite gestures or a pointer, as well as a whistle or clicker if his hearing is still good.

Of course if you do have concerns about your elderly dog's eyesight then have him checked by the vet, as there are conditions that will need diagnosis and treatment. The most common age-related change in your dog's eyes is called 'nuclear sclerosis', where the eyes appear cloudy but he can usually still see quite well. This is often confused with the medical condition cataracts, which do affect vision (senile cataracts). Your vet will be able to differentiate between these two age-related conditions of the eye by using an ophthalmoscope, and will recommend appropriate treatment.

The windows of the soul

Looking into your dog's eyes is not just for working out how well he can see you; it is a useful way of assessing his state of health and vitality as a whole. It has been said that the eyes are the health barometers of the entire body. Indeed, the ancient Chinese believed that the mental and emotional state of the individual (their shen) was reflected in their eyes. So have a good look into your elderly dog's eyes. Are they still sparkling with life, or are they dull and confused?

Hearing

There comes a point in the ageing process when selective hearing – where your dog can hear the biscuit tin lid coming off but not his name when called back on a walk – becomes real deafness. This is because the little hairs, called cilia, in the ear canals have become worn out and cannot effectively conduct sound any more. If your dog does seem to be losing his hearing, help him to cope by making your visual signals more obvious and encouraging him to link your gestures with routine events. This will be like having a special sign language between you. Using lights to signal to your deaf dog can also be useful. For example, using a torch to signal to him to come back in from the garden at night.

Noise phobias

You should also be aware that your dog may become more sensitive to certain noises as he loses his hearing with age, for example becoming scared of thunder or fireworks or jumpy at certain sounds in the house. This can be due to the loss of his mid-range hearing capacity, so that loud noises or sounds at a certain pitch seem sudden and strange and hence frightening. Dogs with loss of hearing can still sense vibration, so clapping your hands or stomping your feet can help to alert him that you are trying to communicate with him. Don't forget that your aged dog will have been picking up on non-audible clues such as your facial expressions and body language for years as part of the way he understands what you are telling him, so he will be less disadvantaged than we might imagine by losing his hearing. The sense of touch will become an even more valuable way of communicating and bonding with your elderly dog, as his hearing and sight begin failing. Regular massage, and even just a gentle but reassuring pat or stroke will help your old dog feel less lonely and anxious. In Traditional Chinese Medicine it is the kidney energy (qi) that is deficient in old age. This is the energy that fuels the sense of hearing and keeps the bones strong and healthy. Therefore it is no surprise to the Chinese doctors when old animals become deaf and suffer from arthritis, because according to their understanding of the ageing process these phenomena go hand in hand. So using acupuncture as a treatment for arthritis can have the added benefit of helping with your dog's hearing.

Smell

This may be the one sense that still works well for your old friend when the others are fading fast. The part of the dog's brain that is concerned with smell contains over 125 million sensitive receptors, which is forty times bigger than the equivalent area in the human brain. This is why dogs are able to discriminate odours at concentrations almost 100 million times lower than we can. No wonder that your elderly dog has such a good time ambling around sniffing on his daily strolls; he is picking up on all the neighbourhood canine gossip from the scents left on every lamp-post and blade of grass. Harnessing his incredible sense of smell can also be a helpful way of rousing or getting the attention of your dog if he is completely blind and deaf. By holding your hand in front of his nose he will quickly become aware of you by your scent. You can even work on using a kind of 'scent' sign language with him. Touch and smell are two senses that you can really harness for communication with your elderly dog.

BEHAVIOUR CHANGES

It is often difficult or impossible to pin down the reasons why old dogs seem

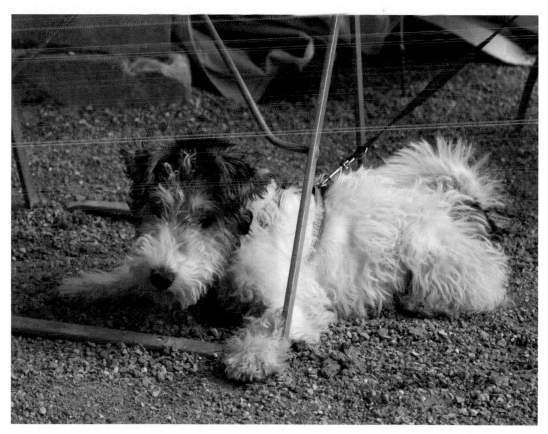

This old chap still takes a keen interest in what's going on.

anxious, unhappy, confused and forgetful, or just not themselves. This is because there are so many parts of growing old that have an impact on how they feel and behave. Loss of brain function is natural in most dogs by the time they reach around sixteen years old, and in some dogs this happens much earlier. Typical behaviour includes disorientation and confusion, changes in how he gets along with other members of the family, people as well as other pets, and sometimes a loss of house-training and alterations in his sleep/wake patterns. Your elderly dog may seem to bark and whine or pace around for no apparent reason, and be restless all night, yet sleep all day. He may snap or growl at you when you go to touch him. He may wait at the wrong side of the door for you to open it for him. He may stare into space or seem forgetful about why he's gone outside or come into a room. Of the different causes of age-related behaviour change, one of the most important factors to consider will be pain. Is your dog uncharacteristically snappy or touchy because he is suffering long-term pain? There is also the deterioration of his sight and hearing, which could be making him feel more vulnerable and anxious. Equally he may actually be showing symptoms related to ageing of the brain itself, a condition called 'Canine Cognitive Dysfunction', which can be compared to senility or Alzheimer's in people.

By looking carefully at how your old dog is behaving, you should be able to see what it is that mainly bothers him. Is it his painful joints or his deteriorating senses? Or does he seem to be losing his marbles? By identifying the most likely underlying cause for your dog's behaviour changes you will able to address them in the most appropriate way. So don't just assume that if your dog no longer gets up to greet you, or fails to respond in his usual way to a knock at the door, it's because he's lazy or uninterested. It may well be because he feels too sore to move, or is confused and disorientated and cannot recognize you due to the onset of senility. Curing these conditions is not usually possible, as they are all just part of the natural ageing process. However, by understanding why they are more likely to occur and how to manage the symptoms (and in some cases slow their progression), you can make sure your old friend doesn't have to turn into the 'grumpy old man' of the dog world.

Chronic pain

When dogs are in pain they will try and protect their achy body from being poked and prodded or, worse still, bumped into. Your dog may make a low growl or curl his lip to tell you that he doesn't want you to touch him because it is painful. This may be for even such a minor thing as clipping his lead on, or giving him a gentle stroke on his head. It may equally be reflected in his fearful and aggressive responses to rowdy or overly enthusiastic dogs in the park, as he is afraid of being hurt and knocked over. Such responses are not innately bad-tempered; they are just painful. Dogs that are feeling sore will be reluctant to move or get out of their beds to go to the toilet, let alone on a walk. This is a sorry state to be in; if your dog is showing any of these signs, such as uncharacteristic aggression, unwillingness to move, or wetting his bed, he should be checked over at the vet's straight away. As well as providing the appropriate treatments to help relieve his pain, there are ways of making your dog's life at home easier.

Firstly, provide him with a retreat, a den or a resting area where he can nap undisturbed. This is especially important if you have a busy household where there is a lot going on. For example, children and younger dogs running about can be quite overwhelming for a frail dog that can't get out of the way as quickly as he needs to. You can also do daily TTouch on your achy, arthritic dog to help relieve muscle spasm, pain and tension in his body (see Chapter 1). While most dogs that have been well socialized and have good awareness and communication skills will be able to read the signs in your aged dog and know to be gentle around him, not all dogs have this sensitivity. Therefore it is better to be safe than sorry and to walk your elderly dog in places where you are less likely to encounter big groups of rowdy dogs. The same attention goes for making sure that friends and family, as well as the stranger in the park and the vet, realize that your dog may be sensitive to touch and slow in his awareness, and so should be gentle and approach him slowly.

Confusion

As the elderly dog's senses deteriorate, so does his awareness of his surroundings. Since he can't see or hear so well, he will be less sure of what is going on around him. This makes the ageing dog more attached to the stability in his life, his routine, his home and people he knows. He will like things to be done in the same way and at the same time every day, and for everything to stay exactly as it has always been – just like the archetypal 'grumpy old man'. Let's be honest, at this stage pandering to his funny ways and habits is probably (where reasonable) the best way of keeping your old dog happy. Keeping his bowls and beds in the same

---

HOW TO SPOT SIGNS OF CHRONIC PAIN

Signs that your dog is in ongoing pain and discomfort can be subtle and easy to miss or mistake for just 'normal' ageing. Dogs can be very stoical when they are feeling discomfort, so you will need to be aware of the following signs that your dog may be uncomfortable, and even in pain:

- Pacing
- Restlessness: constantly settling down and then a little while later getting up again, unable to get comfortable
- Panting, when not hot
- Increased rate of breathing
- More clingy, or more withdrawn
- Uncharacteristic reactions such as intolerance to being touched or moved. Any unexplained, out-of-character reaction
- Licking at a joint or another area of the body.

---

place and sticking to his routine as much as possible will make life more settled for your elderly dog. This is why moving house and redecoration or renovations take more of a toll on your older friend than it would do a youngster. Bach flower essences are excellent natural remedies for helping to balance negative emotions into their positive counterparts. They are especially well suited for use in elderly dogs because of their very gentle action and the way that they can treat these subtle but painful emotional upsets that old age can bring.

BACH FLOWER REMEDIES FOR YOUR ELDERLY DOG

Rock water is a Bach flower essence that helps your dog with the rigidity of being stuck in his ways. Beech is used for intolerance, for example of young playful dogs or a new puppy. Impatiens is used for the pain and grumpiness that is associated with inflexibility. White Chestnut helps address the restlessness and pacing that can be a feature of animals in chronic pain, usually at night. Finally, Cherry Plum is an essence indicated when there is a loss of control, again useful for the restlessness and circling and loss of sanity that can cause the old dog distress. (Dosage and use of Bach Flower Remedies are covered in Chapter 1.)

Anxiety

Research shows that elderly dogs have increased levels of stress hormones in their body, even when resting. This anxiety and over-attachment or clinginess can manifest itself as 'separation anxiety' in dogs that previously never minded being left on their own. Behaviour changes such as this can often go hand in hand with the feelings of confusion described above. There are several effective complementary therapies to help these dogs feel more secure. Using one of the TTouch body wraps on him when he is left on his own provides a feeling of security and protection (like swaddling clothes for babies). Another way of helping your dog to feel less anxious in his old age is to make sure that he has a den or retreat to go to. This should be somewhere snug and secure, such as a cosy

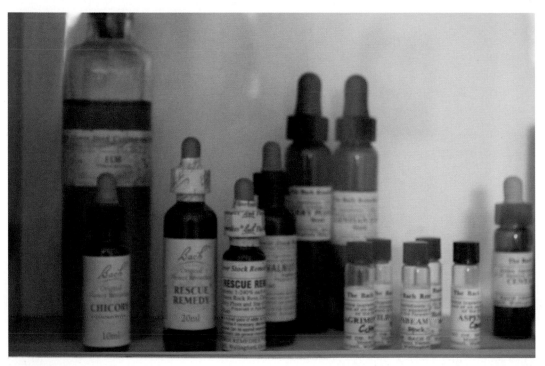

Bach Flower Remedies are useful for elderly dogs.

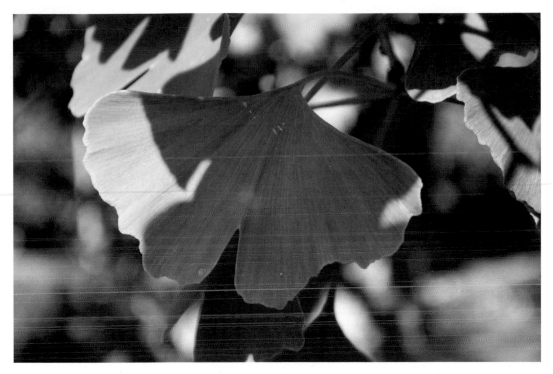

Ginkgo biloba is the key herbal remedy for brain ageing.

spot under a table or in the corner of a room, anywhere he feels enclosed and protected. Another pet as a companion for your elderly dog is one of the best ways of helping him to feel relaxed and safe. Unfortunately, this is not a recommendation to get a bouncy new puppy, as this would be too much for him to cope with. Nurturing him with love and a sense of security will be key to a contented old age for your dog.

Canine cognitive dysfunction

Canine cognitive dysfunction is an age-related degenerative disease of the nervous system of dogs. It has many similarities to dementia and Alzheimer's in people. Dogs with canine cognitive dysfunction (CCD) show many of the signs already described in this section, namely confusion, anxiety, disorientation, loss of house-training, lack of interest, and depression. For example, your dog may ask to go into the garden and then seem to have forgotten what it was he went out there for. Or he may wander aimlessly around the house, bark for no apparent reason, or cry at night. These signs that your dog seems to be losing his marbles indicate that he is likely to be suffering from CCD. However reassuring it may be to have a label for it, this is an irreversible and progressive disorder without a simple 'fix'. The best hope of any treatment will be to slow the progression, and it is believed that in some less advanced cases it may be possible to re-engage some mental function. Ways

HERBAL REMEDIES FOR THE AGEING BRAIN

Ginkgo biloba is one of the oldest plant medicines on earth. With the trees living to 1,000 years, no wonder it is the herb of choice for treating the symptoms of ageing. It improves blood flow, and hence oxygenation, to the brain and also enhances nervous system function. Other herbs that can be helpful for dogs that are displaying signs of brain dysfunction include Gotu kola, another nerve tonic which is said to increase mental clarity, and also peppermint. Nutritional supplements used to help in cases of CCD include Phosphatidylesrine, a major lipid in the brain. Treatment with this essential fatty acid (derived from soya) is believed to increase memory and learning.

and a radio always playing in another. This will make it easier for your elderly dog to know where he is. Another sad consequence of this condition is that your companion may even suffer from an alteration in his moods and personality. The causes and exact mechanisms of how this condition affects the nervous system of aged dogs is as yet unknown and cannot be explained by modern Western medicine. The Ancient Chinese, however, recognized the signs and described this process as a disturbance of the Shen, which is a term for the mind and spirit. The main aim of treatment of CCD is to enhance blood flow, and hence oxygen delivery, to the brain. Of the complementary medicines used for this condition the best-known is the herb Ginkgo biloba (see box). Finally, a senior diet with plenty of antioxidants (especially vitamin E) is another important mainstay of the supportive treatment for ageing dogs suffering signs of CCD.

The second puppyhood

In many respects there are similarities between caring for a puppy and caring for an elderly dog. For both ends of the spectrum it is clear that they benefit from a calm and consistent approach towards their everyday care. Old dogs, like puppies, need more nurturing and support than confident, youthful dogs. Games and activities are something else that has shared importance between young and old. While he still needs a lot of rest and will sleep a lot, try and keep your elderly dog's zest for life alive by continuing to engage him in the activities or outings he used to enjoy. Asking him to perform for a treat (give paw, for example) or rolling a ball along the carpet a little way for him to retrieve will keep his spirits up. If he can no longer get out to chew or sniff

to manage CCD in your dog include avoiding changes in the house that could lead to disorientation; sticking to a daily routine; and making sure he has a comfortable, secure bed that he can easily locate. Because shock and stress are also believed to be possible trigger factors, unnecessary events such as medical interventions or spells in kennels should also be avoided with elderly dogs. The more ways that you can help him to navigate his way around his home, the better for your dog. By increasing the number of clues, using sound, smell and feel to help him know which room he is in, the more grounded and secure he will feel. For example, use certain carpets or floor tiles in different places, have a certain fragrance in one particular room at the grass or plants he used to enjoy, why not pick them for him so that he can still enjoy them from his bed? These kinds of caring, loving gestures will make the world of difference to the enjoyment and fulfilment your old dog gets out of his life. Although he will generally benefit from a quiet life, your old friend mustn't become a total recluse, and will usually enjoy seeing familiar people and dogs that he knows. This will help him retain his social skills, sense of worth and confidence. Despite failing eyes and ears, your dog will understand if you are giving him one-to-one time and gently using your hands to stroke and heal him. He will pick up on the kind, nurturing energy that you are offering him. Finally, it is recognized that stress has a greater impact on older animals. So getting a new puppy if your elderly guy is already showing signs of struggling with the ageing process is not a good idea. If you are looking to get his replacement lined up ahead of time because you don't want to be without a dog, it is far better to do this while your older dog is still mobile and in good shape. This will mean that he can get the most out of the young puppy too, showing him the ropes and acting as a guide and 'wise old friend'. However, he will still have enough energy to move away and show tolerance if the ear-tugging or rough and tumble become too much for him.

MOBILITY AND ARTHRITIS

How to ease aches and pains

Arthritis is the inflammation of joints, from the Greek *arthro-*, joint and *-itis*, inflammation; it causes pain and a reduced range of movement. The arthritis of the older dog is also known as 'osteoarthritis' or 'degenerative joint disease', and is a common age-related condition. The dog's joints become stiff and painful after a lifetime's wear and tear and the degeneration of the protective cartilage cushioning of the joint surface. Dogs that have had increased pressure on their joints due to agility, work or, most commonly, obesity, will be prone to developing arthritis at a younger age. Symptoms can vary hugely, from just the occasional stiffness when your dog first gets up to severe lameness that affects his ability to walk at all. When it comes to arthritis, prevention is much better than cure. The mainstay of conventional treatment is symptomatic pain relief and slowing the progression of the joint degeneration. Holistic therapies, on the other hand, such as TCM acupuncture, aim to address the underlying imbalances as well as easing the pain. Keeping your dog's weight down and making sure he has plenty of regular exercise as he gets older will be helpful. Going out for several ten or fifteen minute walks around the block will be more beneficial for maintaining your dog's mobility than a one-hour amble where he spends more time sniffing the bushes than actually using his legs.

A vicious cycle

Be aware that when old-age aches and pains start to affect your dog this can be the start of a vicious cycle of rapidly deteriorating mobility. As the walks stop, his weight will increase, his muscles waste and his joints get even stiffer and more painful, making the prospect of a walk even less likely. Keeping your dog's muscles in good shape is important not just to allow him to move about, but also because they play a key role in protecting his joints. If the muscles are wasting away, then his knees and hips will have

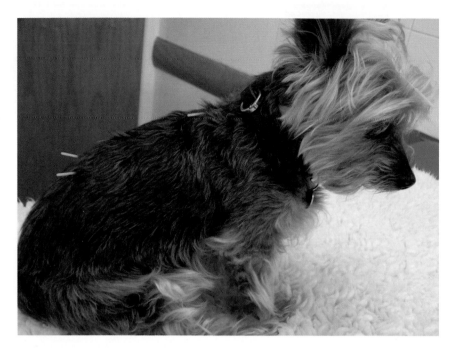

Elderly dogs can benefit from regular acupuncture.

less support and he will be at greater risk of injury, especially if he is also overweight. Fortunately there are a wide range of complementary treatments and nutritional supplements that are highly effective for treating musculoskeletal conditions in dogs. Using these therapies, often alongside a gentle, non-weight-bearing exercise such as hydrotherapy, should keep your old dog in fine physical form for as long as possible.

Acupuncture

This is a well-known complementary treatment for aches, pains and stiffness and is commonly used to treat arthritic dogs. Because it is a holistic therapy, acupuncture is more than just a form of pain relief; it can enhance your dog's overall well-being by boosting appetite, regulating sleep patterns, and supporting liver and kidney function. Acupuncture also stimulates the immune system,

another advantage of this form of treatment for the geriatric dog. In the winter, if your dog is really feeling the cold, then the acupuncturist may use moxa, a Chinese herb, to heat the needles and bring warmth deep into the body. As an all-round tonic for the ageing dog, acupuncture is a holistic treatment that is hard to beat, working well either as the sole therapy or alongside some of those listed below. (For more information *see* Chapter 1.)

Conventional medications

If your dog is suffering pain with his arthritic joints your vet may well put him onto an anti-inflammatory medication to relieve the symptoms. By reducing the inflammation around the problematic joints your dog will be able to exercise with less pain and so maintain strength and general fitness. There are various types of anti-inflammatory drugs used for arthritis, but most common are the non-steroidal anti-inflammatories (NSAIDS). These are usually tablets or liquids given daily over the long term, or they may just be required as a few doses to manage a 'flare-up'. Although they are highly effective as a painkiller, the side effects and the fact that they are just alleviating the symptoms are the limiting factors for using NSAIDS as the sole way of managing arthritis in an elderly dog. With the wide range of complementary medicines and therapies on offer, your dog should be able to benefit from an integrated approach to treatment.

Chiropractic treatment

This is a physical manipulation technique that helps to realign the spine and has an important role in the treatment of dogs suffering from arthritis (*see* Chapter 1).

Herbal medicine

There are several herbs that have a long history of use for the treatment of arthritis (*see* Chapter 1).

Turmeric This Indian herb has the active constituent Curcumin, well documented as having anti-inflammatory and antioxidant properties. It is commonly used for arthritis. A pinch on your dog's food daily is fine.

Boswellia This herb is well known as a natural anti-inflammatory and is now being included in some of the proprietary mobility products along with glucosamines and chondroitin.

Devil's claw This is a traditional South African herb used for arthritis, as well as for digestive complaints, and may be a tonic for older animals with flagging appetites.

Homeopathy

There are a handful of homeopathic remedies well indicated for use in arthritis. Because homeopathy works by matching your dog's individual symptoms to the particular action of the remedy, selecting the right one will depend on your careful observation as well as knowledge of the remedies (*see* Chapter 1).

Rhus Tox One of the most commonly prescribed remedies for arthritis. This is for dogs that are stiff when they first get up after a long rest but ease up after walking around for a bit, and are much affected by the damp.

Rhus Tox, Ruta and Arnica (RRA) This is often used as a combination remedy called RRA. Rhus Tox is used along with Arnica and Ruta, two other remedies helpful for treating muscle and ligament strains and sprains.

Bryonia Used for symptoms of arthritis that are much better for resting and worse for warmth (the opposite to Rhus Tox). When this remedy is indicated, your dog may lie on the affected side so as to keep the painful part of his body as still as possible.

Hydrotherapy

Swimming is a gentle, non-weight-bearing form of exercise that is excellent for keeping the arthritic dog in trim. It maintains his muscle tone and general fitness. It also stimulates his interest and enthusiasm in life, giving him a serotonin boost (like the 'high' we get after exercise). Hydrotherapy is especially useful when used in conjunction with treatments that provide pain relief, such as acupuncture. This is because your dog will be able to move his limbs more freely without it hurting and thus get more benefit from swimming. With the buoyancy of the water supporting his weight, hydrotherapy will encourage your dog to use his limbs properly, getting the greatest range of movement from each of his joints. This way he will rebuild as well as maintain his muscle strength and limb function in a much gentler and more effective way than would be possible on land. Hydrotherapy also plays an important part in weight-control programmes for obese dogs.

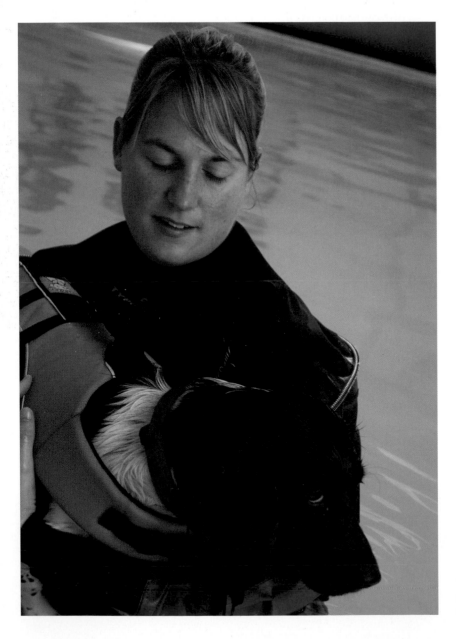

This dog is enjoying hydrotherapy.

Massage and acupressure

It is a natural reaction to want to give your dog a rub if he appears to be in pain and stiff. There really isn't anything fancy or special about massaging your dog, it's as easy or complex as you want to make it. You can simply follow your instincts and let your hands and fingers guide you to work on his sore areas, or you can learn some of the healing manipulative techniques such as massage, TTouch and acupressure. The simplest approach to start with is a gentle but firm massage all over, but concentrating along your dog's spine, from head to tail and along each limb down to his feet. This will help to get his circulation going and ease him into action first thing in the morning. It will also help to alleviate stiffness by moving the qi along the main meridian pathways. As well as a quick rub when he first gets up, a more complete, all-over body massage will be a lovely treat for your older dog to enjoy every day. Of course, if your dog does not want to be touched, or if you find any sore or painful areas, then he should be checked over at the vet's and may well be in need of an acupuncture or chiropractic treatment.

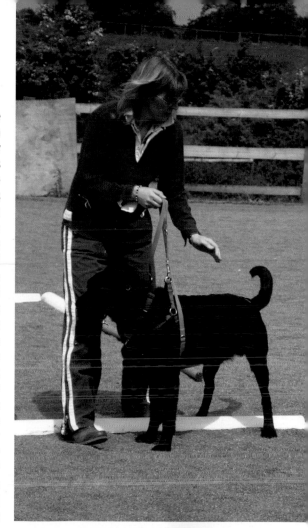

Ground work techniques can help with coordination.

Tellington Touch and ground work

Tellington Touch is different from just ordinary massage (*see* Chapter 1), and is often done together with ground work. This is a way of improving your dog's coordination and body awareness through exercise over and around certain obstacles. Ground work is useful for dogs that tend to trip and stumble, as it helps them to concentrate and be aware of where they are placing their feet. You can easily incorporate these ideas into your dog's everyday walks, by taking him in gentle zig-zag patterns or over different surfaces such as woodchips or sand instead of just on grass or along the road. These techniques help to bring your dog's awareness to his feet and should make him more coordinated and less likely to trip or stumble.

Supplements for arthritis

With an ever-growing array of supplements for the arthritic dog it has become increasingly important to understand how they work and what they contain. Those most commonly used in arthritis, namely glucosamines, are all covered in detail in Chapter 7.

THE SENIOR DIET

Obesity is one of the biggest problems in senior dogs. As well as making it much more difficult for your old friend to get around on his arthritic legs, being overweight affects his heart and general state of health. Therefore it is vital to be aware that as he slows down and becomes less active he will need fewer calories in his daily rations. However, it's not as simple as just feeding him less; your elderly dog actually needs a different, more nutrient-dense food because his ageing body is less efficient at getting all the essential goodness from it. His need has gone up to meet the demands of a lifetime's wear and tear and the ongoing degenerative processes, and to support his weakened immune system. A senior diet should reflect these specific needs by containing high-quality ingredients that are easily digestible and rich in nutrients and vitamins. This diet should consequently contain fewer toxins, thus putting less strain on the liver and kidneys and easing the ageing body's workload. Because the senior diet is more energy- and nutrient-dense, it can be fed in smaller quantities, to match the reduced appetite of the older dog. His digestive system will also be more sensitive as he gets older, making it particularly important not to make any abrupt changes to his diet because of the risk of tummy upsets. This more delicate digestive tract is another

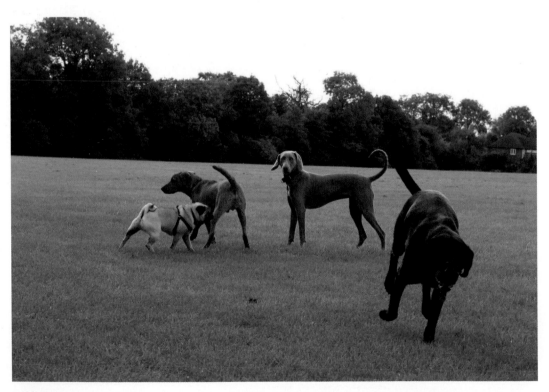

Elderly dogs may prefer to be walked on their own, away from the rough and tumble of a group walk.

reason why senior dogs are fed a more easily digestible diet. This can be either home-cooked or a commercial food that has high-quality, and hence easily digestible, constituents. The more additives and complex, unnatural ingredients in the food, the greater will be the workload on your dog's digestive system.

According to Traditional Chinese Medicine, older dogs should always have their food cooked. As well as helping with digestibility, warming the food will enhance its aroma and stimulate your dog's appetite. If grains are used in the senior dog's diet they should be pre-soaked and thoroughly cooked. Enzymes are the part of the digestive juice that helps to break down the foodstuffs into the building blocks that the body can use. Probiotics are the friendly bacteria in your dog's intestinal system that also play a vital role in digestion and provide essential vitamins in the body. Therefore by adding an enzyme or probiotic supplement to his diet you can help boost your dog's digestive system, helping him get the most out of his food. Finally, the senior diet needs to be rich in antioxi-dants. These are present in all healthy, fresh, natural foodstuffs, but can also be given as supplements in their own right. Antioxidants help combat the everyday signs of ageing, so are a particularly important addition to the elderly dog's diet. Most good-quality nutritional supplements will contain a base of enzymes and probiotics, as well as multivitamins and antioxidants (see Chapter 7). Adding certain herbs to his daily rations can also be of benefit to the older dog.

In summary

Because every dog will age in his own way, with different parts of his body needing support at different times, you may every so often have to alter his diet to meet these changing needs. Therefore evaluating his individual health status by regular vet checks and blood tests will alert you as early as possible to any organ systems that need particular support. Of course, in the ideal world your dog would have had a natural diet throughout his life, ensuring that his organ systems are in good order when he reaches old age, having been spared the lifetime effects of rendered meat and artificial chemical overload.

AT THE VET'S

Senior health checks

Because in relative terms a dog ages more quickly than we do, a twice-yearly health check for him will be like a four-yearly one for us. These senior health assessments are important because the normal signs of old age such as slowing down, lethargy, fussy appetite and stiffness need to be differentiated from the early signs of a disease condition. Your vet will be able to manipulate and

---

HERBAL TONICS FOR THE AGEING DOG

Dandelion and burdock root are mild liver tonics, helping to increase the flow of bile and aid digestion. Milk thistle is another well-known liver support, and as this is the major organ involved in processing drugs, it is an especially useful herb to use if your elderly dog is on daily medications. Finally, spirulina and other blue-green algae are an excellent tonic for supporting the elderly body.

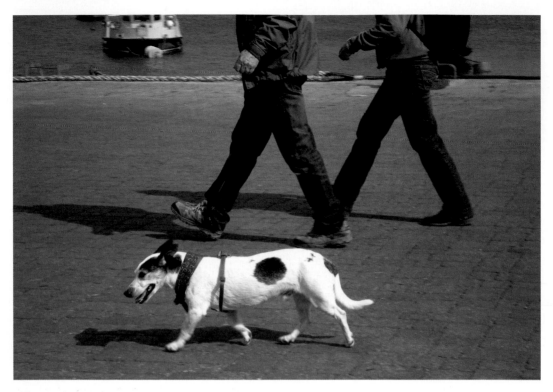

Visits to favourite places are important for elderly dogs.

palpate your dog all over, checking for any worrying lumps or bumps and assessing the range of movement of his joints. He will also listen to your dog's heart and lungs to make sure that his cardiovascular system is still working well. Your dog will also be weighed, because weight loss can be an indicator of underlying disease, as can any significant alterations in his drinking habits or appetite. Your vet will usually offer a blood test and may also run a urine screen to help him to assess how your dog's internal organs are working.

Diagnostic tests and treatment options
Due to the great range of diagnostic tests and procedures now commonplace in

NATURAL SIGNS OF AGEING VERSUS ILLNESS

With natural ageing there is a slowing down of your dog's pace of life. If he is not given special attention and cared for in his old age he can start to feel depressed and lethargic and will stay in his bed more and may no longer want to eat or show interest in his food. However, these are also signs that your dog may be unwell. Therefore it is important that you have him checked over by the vet, as they will be able to differentiate between illness and the normal signs of ageing.

veterinary practice, you can sometimes be faced with a difficult dilemma for your elderly dog. This is especially the case if what he is suffering from is, to all intents and purposes, the effects of old age. Is it fair to put your elderly dog through extensive diagnostic procedures or operations that would involve a stay in hospital? If you are in this position, the best advice will be to consider how your dog would be likely to cope with this, and to discuss with your vet how the results would affect the outcome of his treatment. If you don't think that the diagnostic tests would upset him too much, and indeed if getting the diagnosis is crucial to a highly effective treatment, then it clear that it would be beneficial for your dog to have them. However, if you have no intention of putting your aged dog through an operation, or equally if the thousand-pound scan will not alter the treatment that you can give him, then it is a more difficult decision.

SAYING GOODBYE

Unlike us humans, your dog does not live his senior years in anticipation of death, he just gets on with life as best as he can. However, when your companion does enter the last phase of life it is an agonizing time as an owner, because it is your responsibility to decide when the time is right. Euthanasia is usually the humane course of action where the prognosis is hopeless or where the continued life of your dog would be painful or undignified for him. Although there are no hard and fast rules, it is generally always a question of 'quality of life' – weighing up the amount of pleasure your dog still gets out of life, with the degree that he struggles with physical or mental deterioration. It is often hard to appreciate the overall trend of his quality of life when you are with your dog every day, so it can help to keep a daily record. If his condition seems to vary from one day to the next, as it often does in elderly pets, keeping a daily note of whether he has had a good day or a bad day helps you to see the bigger picture over a few weeks. It is also important to talk it over with your vet (you don't have to have your dog with you), so that you can be sure in your own mind exactly what his problems are, his likely prognosis and the progression of the condition. You can also discuss the options for when it comes to having him put to sleep.

Letting go

This means accepting that you have to have your dog put to sleep. This is a mutual process between you and your dog. Not only do you have to accept that it is time, your dog also has to know that you accept his going. Animals do sense when you are in denial about their death and are effectively holding onto them for your own need. If you are having difficulty coming to terms with the fact that your dog is at the end of his life, talk to him and tell him why you are unhappy and ask him whether he feels that it is his time to pass away. Of course it is not the words out loud that matter, it is the sense of a quiet, intuitive communication between you that is important. Engage with him and be open to what he may communicate to you. He may say that it's his time to go and he wants your permission, or it may not yet be the time. Buddhists understand that dying involves one's consciousness departing the body. Normally, when death comes naturally (rather than through euthanasia), the last few days of life are an important preparation for death and the transition of one's consciousness. Therefore, in order to give your dog's consciousness time to prepare, whether you believe it's for the next life or simply to end this one, talk to him or otherwise communicate that you are arranging for him to be put to sleep in a few days' time. This will help you both prepare for letting go, he to life and you to your old friend.

Euthanasia

When the day comes, you can either take your dog into the surgery or have him euthanased at home. By making the arrangements in advance you will be left with the peace of mind of knowing that your dog enjoyed a fulfilled life in which he had love and respect right up until the last moment. In most cases, where possible, it is obviously a more pleasant experience for you as well as for your dog to arrange for the vet to do a home visit. This way he will be less anxious, will not have to travel in the car and can stay in familiar surroundings. However, if you do have to have it done at the surgery, choosing the first appointment of either the morning or the afternoon session will often mean that you are less likely to have to wait. Euthanasia itself is usually from a lethal injection given into the front leg. The vet will normally have to clip a little of the fur and is likely to have a nurse helping to hold your dog. Staying with him while he is put to sleep will be a great comfort and reassurance for your dog. It may also help if you speak to him and stroke him while the vet is putting him to sleep. Hearing your voice and feeling your touch will let your dog pass away peacefully, feeling loved and cared for.

It is important that you remember your dog in a way that is special to his memory. So whether this is by scattering his ashes in the meadow or woodland that he most loved to romp in, or burying him in a favourite spot and planting a tree, it is a memorial to him.

Bereavement

Other pets in your household will undoubtedly be affected by the loss of their companion. In fact you may have noticed them acting differently towards your elderly dog days or even weeks before he was put to sleep, as they sensed something was wrong. So in their own way they may during this time have been making their peace with him and saying goodbye. It is important for these pets to have the opportunity to see and sniff the departed dog's body after he has died. This way they will be better able to understand and process the fact that he is no longer around and come to a more peaceful acceptance. Giving them the homeopathic remedy called Ignatia, for loss and sudden grief, is another way of helping them to recover. In addition, the use of Bach Rescue Remedy is beneficial for the shock and sadness. If you are grieving yourself and don't have friends or family to support you, there are national charities such as the Pets Bereavement Trust that offer support and counselling.

SENIOR DOG HEALTH CARE AND COMMON AILMENTS

Each of the following symptoms and conditions are potentially serious in the older dog. Therefore you should always have him checked over by the vet in the first instance before attempting any home treatment. Some other ailments are covered in Chapter 9; arthritis, cataracts and incontinence have been covered earlier in this chapter.

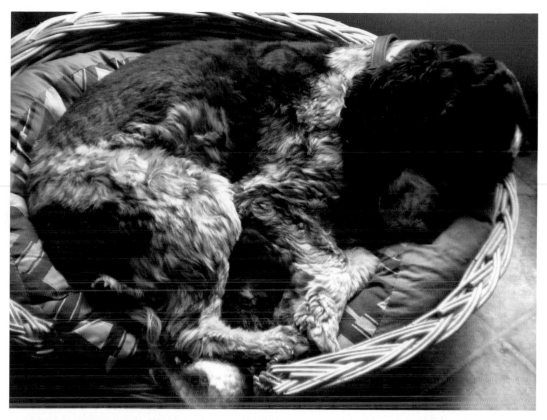

A comfortable place to sleep.

Cancer

There is no doubt that cancer is a disease that is more common in old age. There are many types of cancer and they may not be as obvious as a fast-growing lump that you can readily see. Your vet may need to perform certain diagnostic tests, such as fine needle aspirates or biopsies, in order to diagnose cancer in your dog. How you decide on the right course of action for treatment will vary with every dog and in every different circumstance. In addition to the conventional approaches to treatment, which include chemotherapy, surgery, and even radiotherapy, there are also the complementary therapies to consider. These can be used either as a sole form of treatment or as part of an integrated approach to care.

Kidney disease

Reduced kidney function is one of the most common problems in older dogs. The signs that can alert you to a possible problem with your dog's ageing kidneys include an increase in his thirst, as well as a change in appetite or energy levels, weight loss and sometimes vomiting. Because this is usually a degenerative condition, treatment is aimed at slowing the progression and managing the symptoms, rather than offering a cure. Your dog's diet will be an important way of managing the condition. He will need to be on a diet that has high quality protein, with restricted phosphorus and sodium (salt). Herbal supplements to help support the kidneys include dandelion leaf, which is nature's own diuretic, as well as nettles and cleavers. Deterioration in kidney function can also lead to increased loss of water-soluble vitamins (the B complex and vitamin C), so an increased supply is recommended to compensate for this. The principal homeopathic kidney support remedy is Berberis vulgaris. Acupuncture can also be an effective support treatment for the kidneys.

Liver disease

The liver is the organ of detoxification and after a lifetime's wear and tear it can start to suffer the consequences in old age. However, the liver can of course also be affected by infections, toxic damage and cancer, among several other conditions. The symptoms can range from inappetance and vomiting to abdominal pain and lethargy. Your vet will diagnose the problem and run blood tests. Here again diet plays an important role in supportive treatment. A highly digestible, moderate protein diet is recommended for most liver complaints. Milk thistle is the number one herbal support for the liver, and is part of most proprietary supplements prescribed by vets, along with multivitamins and antioxidants. The homeopathic remedies that are commonly used for liver support include Lycopodium and Chelidonium.

Prostate problems

Painful urination or defecation can be signs of prostate problems in older male dogs. The prostate gland is a gland in the male reproductive system that encircles the urethra (the tube that carries the urine out of the body) and is near the rectum. It tends to enlarge in old age in entire (non-neutered) dogs and can cause them to have problems when urinating or defecating. There may just be age-related enlargement of the gland or, less commonly, it can become inflamed and painful due to infection or cancer. Treatment will usually involve castration as well as medications. Useful supportive complementary therapies for use in age-related enlargement (not for the other causes) include the herbal remedies saw palmetto, hydrangea and nettle. The most important homeopathic remedies for this condition are Sabal Serrulata and Conium. The addition of zinc, vitamin B complex and flax seed oil to the diet is also recommended.

9 HOLISTIC TREATMENTS FOR COMMON AILMENTS

This chapter gives you an overview of the main complementary treatments used for common ailments in dogs – it is not an exhaustive list. With whole books dedicated to this topic, the aim of covering it in just one chapter is to illustrate how complementary medicine can form part of an integrated approach to treatment for your dog. While some of the suggested treatments you will be able to do at home, others will need specialist attention. Preventive health care and holistic management methods are also outlined.

For details of how to use the particular complementary treatments, such as dosing and use of herbal or homeopathic remedies, refer to Chapter 1. Holistic treatments for common ailments in puppies and elderly dogs are given at the end of Chapters 4 and 8 respectively.

Note: If your dog is unwell in any way then he should be taken to the vet's for diagnosis and treatment. The advice given here in no way replaces that of your veterinary surgeon for any sick animal. Finally, it is important that you let your vet know if you are using any form of complementary treatment for your dog, especially if he is on any ongoing medications.

SKIN AND COAT

The condition and general state of his skin and coat are good indicators of the overall health of your dog. As well as its role in protection and sensation, the skin is one of the body's key detoxification organs. According to homeopathic practice, skin symptoms are the first way that the body expresses an imbalance or illness. Nowhere else does your dog's diet and nutritional status reflect itself more clearly than in the state of his skin and

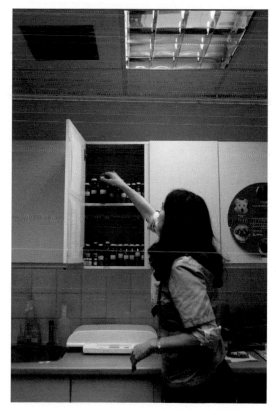

An integrated veterinary practice.

coat. A wholesome, fresh diet is the key to good health and a shiny coat.

Persistent or severe skin and coat complaints will need to be checked by your vet so that they can diagnose the cause of the problem and advise the correct treatment.

Common symptoms

Itching, which in veterinary terms is called pruritis, is the number one symptom of a problem relating to your dog's skin or coat. He may scratch, itch, bite and lick himself all over, or may concentrate on certain parts of his body. Dry skin and dandruff can affect your dog, as can excessively greasy or oily skin. He may lose his fur and develop bald areas or sore, red patches due to excessive and persistent licking, scratching or rubbing at himself.

Routine care for a healthy skin and coat

The most important supplements for maintaining a healthy, shiny, itch-free skin and coat are the essential fatty acids (EFAs). These are the building blocks of the skin, and also have anti-inflammatory action to relieve itching. They are a must-have for any dog with a skin allergy. Give a balanced supplement of omega-3 and omega-6s, found in borage and flax seed oils; or, to make it easier, choose a good quality proprietary supplement, which should also contain vitamin E. It is equally important to keep on top of flea control measures for all dogs (see Chapter 5), but especially for those with flea allergies. Brushing your dog every day is an important part of his routine health care, because as well as keeping him clean it stimulates the skin's oil-producing glands, helping to keep his coat waterproof. Some breeds of dog will need to have their coat clipped, usually at the groom-

ing parlour, every three to four months to stop it getting too long, hot, smelly and unmanageable. Try and minimize your dog's exposure to chemicals by paying attention to the washing powder that you use to wash his bedding. The same goes for household cleaning products, especially carpet cleaners; go chemical-free if you can. This is because when your dog lies on the floor or carpet he will of course be in very close contact with any chemical residues and these may cause irritation to his skin, causing a contact allergy. Feeding your dog a hypoallergenic diet or just avoiding common food allergens such as beef, soya and wheat glutens can be beneficial if he has a skin complaint. Avoiding yeast and wheat is especially important for dogs suffering from Malazzesia, a yeast infection.

Complementary treatments for the skin and coat

Herbal remedies

Burdock, cleavers, nettle and yellow dock are indicated for skin complaints due to their detoxifying action.

Homeopathic remedies

Sulphur is the number one homeopathic remedy for skin complaints. It is used for dogs with itchy, smelly skin that is hot to touch. Arsenicum Album is indicated if the skin is dry and scaly, with the itching being worse at night and where the dog is restless. The dose for these remedies is usually one tablet twice a day for up to five days, using a 12c or 30c potency. Treatment of persistent licking at a particular area (what the vets will diagnose as a 'lick granuloma') can be treated with the homeopathic remedy Ignatia (200c), usually three doses over twenty-four hours. This remedy addresses the underlying anxiety and chronic grief that may be resulting in the excessive licking. Acupuncture can be another useful treatment for this condition.

Treatment of mange

If you or your vet suspect your dog has sarcoptic mange (the most common form of mange), complementary treatment involves building up your dog's immune system via the use of herbs and multivitamin and antioxidant supplements. Garlic can also be used, as mites don't tolerate its rich sulphur compounds. Other herbs to consider for mite infection are lavender, yarrow, Oregon grape, goldenseal and liquorice. They can be used as oils, salves or ointments. Homeopathic remedies include using psorinum 30c once a week for two months.

COMMON CAUSES OF SKIN COMPLAINTS

- Fleas
- Mange
- Allergies
- Secondary bacterial or yeast infection
- Ringworm

Treatment of ringworm

If your vet has diagnosed this fungal infection in your dog (veterinary diagnosis is important as this disease is transmissible to people), the following complementary treatment can be used. Add one or two drops of tea tree oil to a

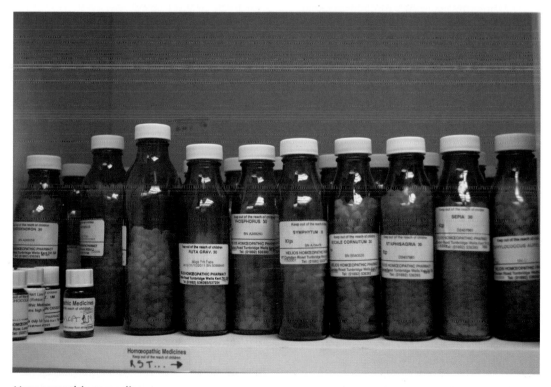

Homeopathic remedies.

little olive oil and the oil from a punctured Vitamin E capsule. This can be applied topically to the lesions, after the hair is clipped away, every day for three to four weeks (take care that your dog does not lick this off). The homeopathic remedy thuja 30c can also be used once weekly during this time.

*Topical treatment for sore
or ulcerated areas*
Clip the fur away from the lesion and then bathe it with a solution of hypercal (a homeopathic antiseptic tincture) or

---

ALLERGIES

Allergies are an exaggerated and unnecessary response of the immune system to a harmless substance, known as an allergen. According to holistic thinking, allergies are caused by an immune system that is out of balance and overreactive. It develops an allergy to whatever potential allergens are around. Thus fleas do not cause a flea allergy; rather the dog is already potentially allergic and fleas are common in his home environment, so he develops an allergy to flea saliva. Once the allergy is present though, the allergens must be avoided as much as possible until the dog's sensitivity can be reduced. If the allergy is to fleas then these must be avoided and good flea control is essential. If the allergy is to foodstuffs then a specific diet is necessary (where the allergen is eliminated). In addition to removal of the allergen, holistic treatment will be through constitutional homeopathic remedies and support of the immune system through nutrition.

---

warm, salty, sterile or boiled water. Soothing aloe vera gel or hypercal cream can then be applied to the area twice daily. An oatmeal compress can also be used; this is soothing and helps to relieve the itch. You can also apply a green tea bag to the area as a cold poultice, as this is full of antioxidants and astringent and so helps to dry the area.

Bathing your dog
Dogs don't need regular baths and bathing them too often strips their skin of its natural oils, leaving them predisposed to skin problems. However, if your dog has rolled in something unsavoury (usually fox excrement) then there is no denying a bath is usually in order. Your dog's skin has a different pH (acidity) to human skin, so it's best to use 'dog' shampoo. For 'routine' washing choose a shampoo according to your dog's coat type and condition. By choosing one that is labelled hypoallergenic you are also usually ensuring that it is free of perfumes and dyes. If possible try and make sure that it is organic (difficult to find), and free of parabens and sodium laurel sulphate (SLS) (these are chemical preservatives and lathering agents that are best avoided). Whichever shampoo you choose, use it very diluted and make sure that you rinse it off well, as residues can aggravate itchiness and cause dry skin. An old-fashioned tip for the rinsing water is to use a cup of chamomile tea with a squeeze of lemon juice for light-coloured dogs, and a sprig of rosemary with added cider vinegar (one tablespoon) for those with a dark-coloured coat.

For itchy dogs
Bath with an aloe and oatmeal shampoo, as this is soothing and cleansing. The aloe also has antimicrobial action, so is

beneficial for mild skin infections. Oatmeal shampoo is easy to make yourself. Just take a handful of oats and place inside a sock or stocking, swish it around in the water to leave a milky residue, and add a few drops of lavender oil. Rinse with fresh water with a few drops of thyme essential oil.

For dogs with dry skin and dandruff
Use moisturizing agents that will help to lubricate, rehydrate and restore the normal skin surface and soften the skin and coat. Use shampoos that are emollients, emulsifiers or humectants, containing active ingredients such as salicylic acid and borage oil.

For greasy coats
A vinegar and water (one third organic cider vinegar and two thirds water) soak for the feet, rinse for the body, or douche for the ears helps reduce yeast.

EARS

Ear problems often go hand in hand with, or are a first symptom of, generalized skin conditions. The ear canal has a delicate lining and contains a fine balance of 'good bugs' (bacteria and yeasts) that become out of balance in ear infections. Breeds with droopy ears or narrow ear canals (such as Spaniels and Bassets) can be prone to ear complaints because little air can get to the ear canal. Thus moist conditions occur where yeasts can proliferate. Dogs such as terriers that actually have hair inside their ear canals can also be prone to problems. Ear infections after swimming, either due to picking up an infection or from excess moisture in the ear canals, can be a problem in some dogs. Getting foreign bodies such as grass seeds stuck in ears

can also happen, particularly during the spring and summer months. Recurrent or ongoing ear problems are usually a symptom of a more deep-rooted disease, requiring more in-depth treatment for lasting cure.

As well as outer ear infection your dog can also suffer from middle and inner ear disease. These are much more serious and will certainly necessitate a visit to the vet's and immediate treatment. It is important never to use any ear-drops or attempt other home treatments in such cases without seeing the vet first.

Due to the wide variety of possible causes, it is important to have any ear condition diagnosed by the vet so that the correct form of treatment can be used.

Common symptoms
Your dog can suffer from symptoms that range from the odd shake of his head to persistent ear irritation where he will scratch vigorously at them. One or both ears may be red, smelly and sore as well as painful. He may have smelly, crusty discharge at the opening to the ear, and your dog may also cry if you touch his ears. If he has persistent or severe head shaking or is holding his head to one side this may be a sign of a foreign body such as a grass seed in his ear, or due to a growth such as a polyp in the ear canal. Your dog can also suffer from swelling to one of his ear flaps, which vets call aural haematomas. These happen when the small capillaries in the ear flap break as your dog shakes his head, usually due to an underlying ear infection. Symptoms of middle and inner ear disease include loss of balance, nausea and disorientation, which are also signs of several other serious illnesses that will equally require rapid veterinary attention.

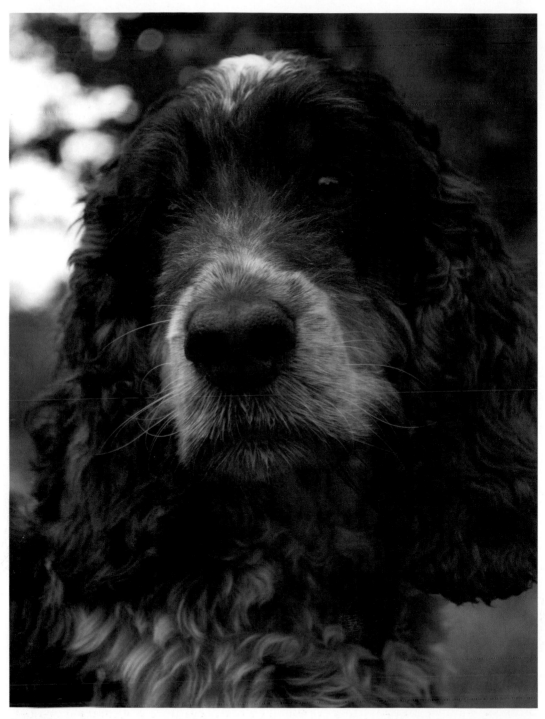

Spaniels can be prone to ear complaints.

Routine care for healthy ears

For routine cleaning of healthy ears use a vinegar and water solution, but never use this in inflamed or sore ears as it will sting. Vinegar acidifies the ear environment and helps to keep bacteria and yeast under control. Use one third organic cider vinegar and two thirds spring water (some people use 50/50). Using a syringe, gently douche the ear canal with one to three millilitres of the solution. This can be used every few weeks, as long-term prevention in dogs prone to infections. It is also useful to help dry the ears after swimming. For waxy ears, apply a few drops of olive oil (or almond oil) into the ear to remove excess wax, wiping away the residue with cotton wool. For dogs that have very hairy ear canals it will be a good idea to gently pluck out a little hair every so often as part of his routine care. You can do this with your fingers, just a very little at once so as not to hurt him. Never use cotton buds in the ear as they can damage and irritate the delicate lining of the ear canals.

Complementary treatments for ear complaints

Ear drops

Take two tablespoons of olive oil and puncture one capsule of vitamin E, mix together and add a few drops of grape seed extract (mullein or garlic can be used instead). This is a good antiseptic mixture and is effective as an anti-fungal and anti-bacterial agent, helping to fight ear infection. Apply a few drops in the ear twice a day for a week, gently massaging the base of the ear after each application. An alternative to this herbal oil is to use a homeopathic hypercal solution to douche the ear; this is more applicable if there is not excessive wax. Always make sure that your

> ### COMMON CAUSES OF EAR COMPLAINTS
>
> - Infection
> - Part of a generalized skin condition
> - Foreign body (such as grass seeds)
> - Ear mites

vet has checked your dog's ears first, as you should never put drops into his ear if he is suffering from middle or inner ear disease.

Homeopathic remedies

Belladonna, 30c, for sudden onset conditions where the ears are painful, red, and hot. Sulphur, 30c, when the ears are hot, with smelly discharge and are part of a generalized skin complaint. Both can be used twice daily for seven days. For swollen ear flaps, where your vet has diagnosed a haematoma, Arnica and Hamamelis, 30c twice daily for up to fourteen days, can be used. This can be given in conjunction with draining and/or ear drops for any underlying infection.

Herbal remedies

You can use herbal remedies such as echinacea, astragalus, goldenseal or Oregon grape root to support your dog's immune system if he has an ear infection. Yarrow or witch hazel can be helpful as external applications for small haematomas of the ear flap, as they help to strengthen capillaries and constrict weak blood vessels.

EYES

Eyes give an important clue to the overall health of your dog, reflecting imbalances elsewhere in his body in the same way that the coat does. They also reflect your dog's spirit and his emotional state, showing whether he is content, anxious or depressed, for instance. Eyes are complicated structures, and problems can affect any part of them from the lids to the clear surface of the eye, the cornea, to the lens or the glands that produce the lubricating tears. Your dog can suffer from simple infections such as conjunctivitis, or he can get foreign bodies such as grass seeds stuck in his eye. Ulceration to the clear surface, the cornea, can also commonly occur due to a scratch from a bramble or an irate cat, for example. Trauma to the cornea can also be caused by friction from an inward turning eyelid (a problem in certain breeds) or a growth on the inner eyelid, more common in older dogs. Your dog can also suffer from persistent eye problems if he has insufficient tears to lubricate them; hence he will be prone to recurrent infections. This is most commonly due to a condition called 'Keratoconjunctivitis sicca' (KCS) or 'dry eye', where your dog's tear-producing glands do not work properly. One of the most painful and potentially serious conditions affecting your dog is glaucoma, where there is an increase in the pressure inside his eye. This can be due to generalized disease in the body or because of localized eye disease. Cataracts may cause opacity of the eye. These develop when the transparent proteins in the lens become cloudy, usually as a result of old age but also with diseases such as diabetes. They are often confused with age-related hardening or 'sclerosis' of the lens, where the cloudiness is like that of cataracts.

You can never be too careful whenever you are dealing with problems in or around the eyes. Seemingly minor symptoms can actually require urgent veterinary treatment in order to save your dog's eyesight. Eyes that become red very suddenly are a true veterinary emergency.

Your vet should examine any eye condition, however mild, straight away.

Common symptoms

Discharge from the corners of one or both eyes is a common symptom of an eye problem. It is usually green or yellow and may affect one or both eyes or go from one to the other. Sore, irritated eyes will usually appear red, with both the conjunctiva and sclera (the white of the eye) being inflamed. Your dog may also paw and rub at his face and eyes if he is suffering from a problem. Cloudiness, excessive discharge, even watery discharge can also spell problems. Similarly, if your dog is squinting or seems uncomfortable in bright light, these are all symptoms of an eye complaint. All of these symptoms require an immediate visit to the vet's. The same is true if you are in any way concerned about your dog's vision.

Routine care for healthy eyes

Make sure that your dog does not have long-term exposure to a smoky environment or air pollution. It is also advisable not to use air fresheners or other household sprays near your dog. One of the reasons why it is not a good idea for him to have his head out of the car window when you are driving is to avoid the problems of airborne pollutants getting stuck in his eyes.

Always check with the vet before using any topical eyewash on your dog.

Complementary treatments for eye complaints
Dietary support
Add a few blueberries or blackberries,

and some yellow and green leafy vegetables, to your dog's diet. These are all rich in beneficial flavinoids, carotenes and antioxidants that are good for ocular health.

Eye drops
A basic eyewash can be made by adding one to two drops of the homeopathic tincture Euphrasia to sterile saline eye-irrigating solution. Bathe the eye twice or three times daily for up to a week.

Herbal remedies
The herb eyebright is supportive for any eye complaint.

Homeopathic remedies
Euphrasia to support any eye complaint. The following remedies are indicated for conjunctivitis: Allium Cepa, where the conjunctiva is red and inflamed, and the discharge is profuse and watery; Argentum Nitricum can be used if the eyes are swollen and bloodshot and the discharge is green; Pulsatilla, if the discharge is bland and creamy, and the conjunctivitis switches from one eye to the other; Sulphur is the remedy of choice for sore, dry eyes where the eyelids are red. These remedies are usually used at a 12 or 30c potency twice daily for a week.

TEETH AND GUMS

Prevention is the best approach when dealing with your dog's dental health. As you'd expect, it is his diet that plays the major role in the state of health of his teeth and gums. Diets that contain fresh meat and vegetables are more effective than sticky, soft diets at preventing the accumulation of tartar and hence the development of gum disease. The abrasive effect of gnawing on raw meaty

COMMON CAUSES OF EYE COMPLAINTS
• Bacterial conjunctivitis
• Corneal ulcer
• Foreign body
• Pressure on the surface of the eye from an in-turned eyelid/growth
• Keratoconjunctivitis Sicca (Dry Eye)
• Glaucoma
• Cataract

bones also helps to strengthen the periodontal ligaments, which hold the teeth in their sockets. Chewing stimulates saliva production, which helps keep the mouth healthy and clean. Inflammation of the gums is called gingivitis and is a response to the plaque on your dog's teeth. If left untreated this will lead to periodontal disease and eventually loss of teeth. As well as his diet, the breed of your dog can also affect his dental health. Dogs with overcrowded dentition, such as the toy breeds or those with malocclusion, will be predisposed to periodontal disease. The other consequence of gingivitis is that the bacteria from the gums circulate around the entire body, and have been linked to systemic conditions such as heart and kidney disease. Your dog's overall health will be compromised because his immune system will be under constant strain having to battle the infection in his mouth.

Common symptoms of dental disease
To assess the state of your dog's teeth and gums gently lift up his lip and have a look. His gums should be a nice healthy pink, his teeth should be fairly white, and his breath not too offensive.

Accumulations of brown tartar, a red line at the gum margin and halitosis are all signs that your dog is suffering from dental disease. If it is severe he may also find it painful when he is eating and his gums may bleed.

Routine dental care

Unless you are brushing your dog's teeth to remove it, or he is on a diet whereby it is mechanically removed in chewing, plaque builds up on your dog's teeth every day. Plaque is invisible, but accumulates to become the hard brown material that we can see, which is called tartar. Plaque can be removed by brushing, tartar can't. Tartar causes inflammation of the gums, gingivitis and periodontal disease, which eventually leads to rotten teeth and tooth loss. Dental chews are not recommended because they usually contain colours, flavourings and other artificial additives and can also be high in calories.

Teeth brushing

Daily tooth brushing is especially important if your dog does not get raw bones to chew on. Get him used to it from a puppy. When you are starting out just massage his gums with your fingers, before introducing a toothbrush. Use toothbrushes designed for dogs, or old human ones, baby ones, or rubber finger brushes; the key thing is that they are soft. You can use an electric toothbrush too if your dog will tolerate the sound. Ask your vet, or the nurse, to give you a demonstration of how to brush your

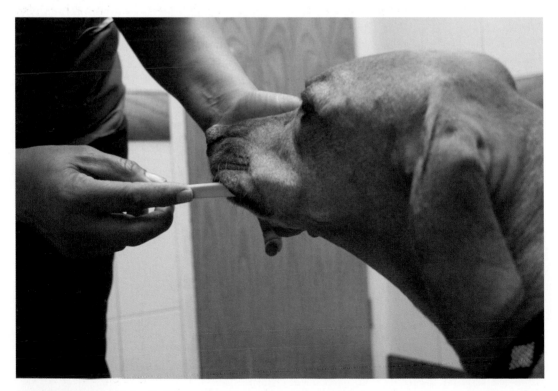

Brushing your dog's teeth is important.

Use a soft toothbrush.

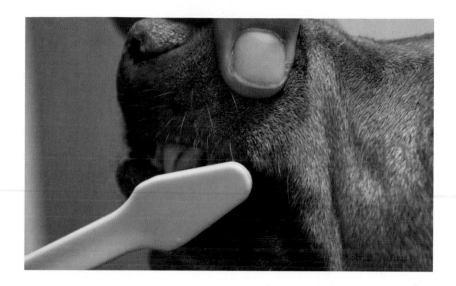

dog's teeth. Start by doing it for just for a few minutes a day and build up. If you make it a habit and follow it with a treat or reward, your dog will soon start to enjoy it. Don't forget that he may require a 'dental' in order to remove severe accumulations of tartar, before you are able to start tooth brushing effectively. Brushing his teeth when he already has gingivitis and periodontal disease will be both ineffective and painful. Choose a dog toothpaste that is free of artificial flavourings and colourings, is low foaming and contains a beneficial herb such as sage oil.

Complementary treatments for dental disease

Diet

Fresh food means healthy digestive processes and sweeter breath. Adding the herbs fennel, peppermint, and especially parsley, to your dog's daily diet can help his breath smell sweeter.

Homeopathic remedies

Arsenicum Album or Phosphorus if the gums bleed easily. Mercurius solibulis for swollen gums with foul odour; use at 30c twice daily for five days. Fragaria is also said to help soften tartar, making it easier to remove; use 12c twice daily for three or four weeks.

Supplements

Antioxidants, vitamins C and E, and especially coenzyme Q10.

Topical

The following can be rubbed directly onto the gums using your fingers or a cotton bud: manuka honey, propolis, sage oil, or bruised fresh sage leaves. Or make up a tincture of Oregan grape, goldenseal, thyme, sage or rosemary. Hypercal solution can be applied to sore gums topically too.

Dentals

If he has severe accumulation of tartar and accompanying periodontal disease, your dog may have to have a 'dental'. This involves a scale and polish, as well as the removal of any rotten teeth, under anaesthetic. After a dental your dog will need to have softer foods for a week or so while his gums are still tender. You can help speed his recovery by giving him Arnica 30c twice daily for three to five days after the dental. Also use a hypercal solution rinse if he has had extractions as this has antiseptic and healing properties. Now, when his teeth are shiny and clean, is the time to begin a new regime of daily brushing. You should also address the way you feed him to optimize the mechanical removal of plaque by natural means. Don't delay though, because your dog's teeth can soon be back in the same state they were before the dental.

THE DIGESTIVE SYSTEM

The digestive system can be affected by stress, anxiety, parasites, infections, food allergies, physical obstructions and the imbalance of intestinal microflora. The role of the digestive system is fundamental to your dog's well-being. If he cannot digest his food properly, this will result in a cascade of other health problems because his nutritional needs are not being met. Many chronic illnesses have their root cause in digestive disturbances. While vomiting and diarrhoea can often be mild and self-correcting, they can also be symptoms of a much more serious complaint. Therefore if you are in any doubt, or if your dog shows any symptoms of abdominal pain or discomfort, is lethargic, off his food, has any blood in his stools, or has vomited several times, then he needs to see the vet. Dogs can quickly become dehydrated from profuse or continued diarrhoea and/or vomiting, hence the need for early veterinary attention if any symptoms are ongoing. In addition, retching, bloating and collapse are all symptoms that indicate your dog requires urgent and potentially life-saving veterinary treatment.

Common symptoms
Dogs are scavengers and hunters by nature, and therefore being able to regurgitate and vomit are important functions for them. In fact dogs do tend to cleanse their own systems every now and then, intuitively inducing vomiting by eating couch grasses, the folk name for which is 'dog grass'. However, if your dog does more than occasionally regurgitate after eating grass, this can be a sign that there is a problem with his digestive system. Vomiting and diarrhoea can occur separately or both symptoms can occur together, it will depend on the cause of the problem. Either symptom can vary from mild to severe, and may occur suddenly or have been ongoing. Colitis is an inflammation of the large intestine, the colon, which results in loose, mucoid stools. Diarrhoea and vomitis can vary greatly in amount, colour and consistency. It is often urgent and your dog may have accidents in the house and overnight. Dogs with a digestive disturbance are also frequently off their food and inappetant.

Routine care for digestive complaints
If your dog has a mild tummy upset resulting in diarrhoea, with no other symptoms, and he is bright and well in himself, then things might resolve by simply skipping his next meal and encouraging rest and recuperation. Always allow access to water. If this is not sufficient you can starve him for twenty-four hours, and then begin feeding him little and often with bland, easily digestible food such as boiled chicken or white fish, and rice. Rice is used as a grain source as it is gluten-free, highly digestible and

ferments less than other grains. It also contains substances that support the cells lining the digestive tract. You can also offer your dog a fluid electrolyte supplement to drink; this is available from the vet's and can help him to stay well hydrated. You can then gradually reintroduce his usual food after a few days, if all is going well.

Complementary treatments for digestive complaints
Herbal remedies
For diarrhoea, slippery elm and plantain can be used to help to firm up the stools. They also contain mucilage, which helps to soothe and protect the intestinal lining. Chamomile, peppermint and ginger are other soothing digestive herbs that can help to relieve nausea and vomiting. They can be given as tinctures or infusions.

Homeopathic remedies
Nux Vomica for diarrhoea and vomiting that is due to overeating or eating rotten or rancid foods. Arsenicum Album if there are traces of blood in the diarrhoea and if the dog seems weak and lethargic. Ipecacuana if there is retching and blood in the vomitis. Podophyllum for diarrhoea that is of sudden onset and

---

COMMON CAUSES OF DIGESTIVE COMPLAINTS

- Scavenging
- Parasites and infections
- Food intolerance – allergy
- Foreign body/physical blockage
- Metabolic or underlying medical complaint

---

profuse, watery and exceptionally offensive. These can all be used at 30c potency twice daily for a week.

Supplements
Kaolin and probiotics to help restore and re-establish the good bacteria in the intestines.

Complementary treatment for travel-sickness
Valerian and skullcap are herbs that can help dogs to sleep in the car, so may relieve car-sickness that is related to anxiety. Giving your dog a few drops of Rescue Remedy before the journey can also help to relax him. The homeopathic remedy Cocculus, 30c, is used for travel-sickness; one dose can be given two to four hours before the journey and another just before travel. It can then be repeated every four hours during the journey. Ginger is the herb most commonly associated with helping to alleviate travel-sickness.

Constipation
Many factors can contribute to constipation, including diet and inactivity. Regular activity helps to maintain regular bowel function. If your dog suffers with chronic constipation then the underlying cause needs to be diagnosed by the vet.

Routine management of constipation
Diet
Fruit and vegetables will increase both the fibre and water content of the diet and be beneficial. Cut down on raw bones in the diet, as too many of these can cause impactions. Encourage water intake and add water to his food. Adding a few tablespoons of cooked pumpkin to your dog's food every day will be helpful. Similarly, add bran or ground flax seed or

psyllium husk to help improve stool consistency.

Exercise and routine

Even a short walk can encourage toileting and increase regularity. Being consistent with timing of feeding and walks will also help your dog's digestive system to function properly.

Complementary treatments for constipation

Acupuncture

Another method of stimulating gut motility in dogs with chronic constipation.

COMMON CAUSES OF CONSTIPATION

- Lack of dietary fibre and moisture
- Obesity
- Medications
- Irritable bowel disease
- Nerve function problem
- Prostate disease (males)

Herbal remedies

Marshmallow root to help to lubricate the intestines.

Homeopathic remedies

Alumina for chronic constipation or Nux Vomica if the constipation has come about after use of medications. Use 30c twice daily for a week.

Supplements

Probiotics and digestive enzymes. Live yoghurt activates the reproduction of the intestinal flora and can also have quick and natural laxative effects.

Flatulence

The most common cause of flatulence is your dog's diet and his digestive processes. Excessive and offensive flatulence indicates excessive fermentation in the bowel and is usually due to his diet being too high in certain foods such as legumes and beans.

Routine management for flatulence

A change of diet may be helpful. Avoid soya, beans, legumes and cabbage. Include a few tablespoons of live yoghurt. The diet should be highly digestible, which means that it consists of good

---

POISONOUS FOODS

Always keep human and animal medicines separate and never give your dog any medicine intended for human use. Keep all medicines in a safe place, out of reach of your dog. The following foods have known toxicity to dogs (this is not an exhaustive list):

- Avocados
- Chocolate
- Garlic in excess – used in moderation, it is a medicinal herb
- Grapes, raisins and sultanas
- Onions
- Some nuts
- Xylitol-sweetened foods

If you know that your dog has eaten any amount of any of these substances, contact your vet straight away. If you have to take your dog to the vet's always take the poison and any remaining packaging with you.

---

quality ingredients, so that there are fewer residues for fermentation in the large bowel. Exercise is also important to stimulate stools and get rid of waste.

Complementary treatments for flatulence
Supplements
Probiotics, digestive enzymes and multi-vitamins, especially B complex.

Eating faeces
This is a complaint called coprophagia, and to a certain extent is part of a dog's normal scavenging behaviour. It becomes a problem if he is doing it all the time. It is most likely that your dog does it as a habit, or due to another behavioural issue. Checking whether your dog just eats his own faeces, or that of other dogs, or even that of other animals, may give you some clues as to the underlying reason he does it. A veterinary check-up may help to diagnose whether there are any underlying nutritional deficiencies or medical reasons causing it, but these are rare. If it is purely a behavioural issue you may need to seek expert advice.

Routine management of coprophagia
In addition to addressing the underlying cause, you can look at your dog's diet. Try changing it; offer him a different type, brand or flavour of food. Anecdotes advise adding pineapple to his food to deter him from eating his own faeces. Adding a multivitamin and mineral supplement, probiotics and digestive enzymes may be of benefit.

Anal gland problems
The anal glands are under the skin on either side of the anus. They produce a scent-like substance that is squeezed onto the faeces during each bowel motion.

Common symptoms
Impacted or infected glands cause your dog to scoot along, rubbing his bottom on the ground. He may also lick at himself because anal gland problems are uncomfortable. If your dog constantly licks his bottom or is irritated, another possible cause will be a food allergy.

Routine management of anal gland problems
Your vet may need to express and empty your dog's anal glands, and will then be able to assess the secretions and check for infection. Your vet will also be able to feel whether there are any abnormalities with the anal glands themselves, such as impaction, thickening or growths.

Diet
Add fibre, such as a spoonful of porridge oats, to bulk up the stools and hence encourage natural emptying of the anal glands.

Complementary treatments for anal gland problems
Herbal remedies
If the glands are infected use garlic and echinacea to boost your dog's immune system and help to combat infection.

COMMON CAUSES OF ANAL GLAND PROBLEMS

- Soft stools and dietary factors
- Irregular bowel movements
- Recent diarrhoea
- Poor muscle tone
- Obesity

Homeopathic remedies
Silica, 30c, can be used twice daily for five to seven days to help with chronically blocked anal glands.

Topical
Apply calendula cream to soothe and heal inflamed areas. Use manuka honey for infected glands.

THE RESPIRATORY SYSTEM

The respiratory system includes the nose, windpipe, bronchial tubes and the lungs, and it is intimately linked with the cardiovascular system. The body uses sneezing and coughing as a way of expelling debris and infectious agents from the respiratory system. It is important not to suppress these symptoms but instead to boost the body's efforts to cleanse the airways. One of the most common causes of a cough in dogs is 'kennel cough' (also called infectious tracheobronchitis). However, a persistent or severe cough could also be a sign of a much more serious condition such as pneumonia, bronchitis or heart disease. Some dogs are more prone to respiratory-system problems due to their anatomy, such as breeds with short noses and an overly long palate, which can sometimes make breathing difficult. Other dogs may suffer from a collapsing windpipe or laryngeal paralysis, both of which can obstruct the normal flow of air. Finally, grass seeds and other small foreign bodies can get lodged up your dog's nose, causing obvious problems.

Due to the wide variety of possible causes, some minor and others very serious, it is important to have any respiratory-system problem diagnosed by the vet so that the correct form of treatment can be used.

Common symptoms
Any change in your dog's normal breathing rate or rhythm is a possible cause for concern, as is any change in his stamina, such as breathlessness on a normal walk. Rapid breathing can be caused by excitement or fear but can also be a sign of pain. Coughing and/or sneezing are further symptoms of a respiratory-system problem. Coughs can differ widely from the dry to the productive, from the intermittent tickle to the persistent hacking. Your dog may remain bright and well, or he may become quiet and weak from coughing. He may also be sneezing and have nasal discharge associated with a cough. If he has temporarily lost his sense of smell, your dog may also be off his food. Nasal discharge from just one nostril, with accompanying discomfort, may indicate the presence of a foreign body lodged up your dog's nose.

Kennel cough
'Kennel cough' (infectious tracheobronchitis) is a highly infectious cough causing a particularly characteristic harsh, hacking sound that is followed by retching. It is the most common cause of coughs in dogs. It is self-limiting, which means it will usually clear up on its own within a few weeks, but it can be debilitating for the very young or the very elderly. Some dogs can remain persistently infectious for a long time after the symptoms have cleared up, which is one of the reasons it is such a common complaint. Drosera and Spongia Tosta are the homeopathic remedies most often indicated for treating kennel cough. The kennel cough nosode (a remedy made from the infectious agent) can be used to dose dogs that have been exposed to kennel cough or are at risk of catching it. These are used at 12c twice daily for five to seven days.

Routine care for the respiratory system
Make sure that the air inside your home is as healthy as possible by opening the windows whenever you can and having houseplants to help keep the air clear and pure. Avoid synthetic air fresheners and of course don't smoke near your dog. If your dog is suffering from a respiratory-system complaint, such as a cough, use a harness instead of a collar and lead to walk him. A collar may exacerbate a sore throat when there is pressure on it from a lead.

Complementary treatments for respiratory-system complaints
Herbal remedies
Liquorice acts as an expectorant, so is helpful in productive coughs. Thyme and garlic can be used for dry coughs such as kennel cough.

Homeopathic remedies
Antimonium Tartaricum for rattly coughs with much loose mucus. Arsenicum Album for asthmatic coughs and Ipeca-cuana for coughing spasms. For watery nasal discharges and sneezing, Allium Cepa is indicated. Kali Bich is the remedy of choice for nasal discharges that are ropey yellow, with crusts to the nostrils

> **COMMON CAUSES OF RESPIRATORY SYSTEM COMPLAINTS**
>
> - Kennel cough
> - Other infectious causes (including lungworm)
> - Physical obstructions to airways
> - Heart disease
> - Airborne allergens
> - Bronchitis
> - Pneumonia

and violent sneezing. These remedies are used at a 12 or 30c potency twice daily for a week.

Acupuncture
Effective at helping to clear the sinuses and boost the immune system.

Supplements
The addition of one teaspoon of manuka honey to your dog's food is both soothing and antimicrobial. It is also a good idea to soak his dry food if he has a cough, making it less irritating for a sore throat.

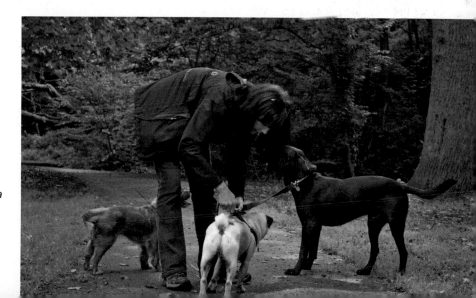

If your dog has a cough a harness may be helpful.

Steam inhalation

To help relieve sinus congestion, let your bathroom fill with steam by running a hot bath or shower, add eucalyptus oil to the water and let your dog stay in there for between five and ten minutes. You can then gently rub and pat over his chest area with a cupped hand to help loosen the mucus via coupage. (Don't do this in conjunction with homeopathic treatment, as the strong scent may antidote the remedy.)

THE HEART

Dogs can suffer from several forms of heart disease, from congenital conditions to degenerative diseases such as those affecting the heart valves. Other forms of heart disease may be secondary to infection from bacteria, viruses or parasites. The symptoms most commonly related to a heart complaint include lethargy, not wanting to exercise, breathing difficulties and coughing, especially when lying down at night. Your vet may also detect irregular heart rhythms when he listens to your dog's heart with a stethoscope, and related symptoms such as fluid in his chest or abdomen.

It goes without saying that if you suspect your dog is suffering from any form of heart condition then the vet should see him straight away. The following suggestions for supportive complementary treatments are to be used under veterinary guidance only, and are not intended as sole forms of therapy in serious conditions.

**Complementary treatments
for heart support**

Acupuncture

Beneficial for heart conditions.

Diet

Use potassium-rich foods such as green leafy vegetables (broccoli and spinach). Consider occasionally adding fresh (organic) heart to the diet too.

Exercise

Keep your dog's weight under control if he suffers from any form of heart condition. Regular gentle exercise is usually beneficial because it will help to oxygenate the body and stimulate the circulation.

Herbal remedies

Hawthorn is the principal heart herb. It helps to improve coronary blood flow, moderate blood pressure and strengthen the heartbeat. Gingko or cayenne are used to help increase circulation to the extremities. Dandelion leaf tea acts as a natural diuretic, helping to rid the body of excess fluid that builds up in cases of congestive heart failure.

Homeopathic remedies

Crataegus is a heart support remedy (derived from hawthorn), used daily at a 6c potency or as a tincture.

Supplements

Omega-3 fatty acids are very good for the heart; fish oils, such as salmon, are rich sources. Vitamin E and selenium are also beneficial. L-carnitine and coenzyme Q10 are other supplements that your vet may recommend.

THE URINARY SYSTEM

The most important job of the urinary system is to get rid of toxic substances and maintain the body's water balance. The kidneys also produce hormones that affect the circulatory system. The bladder is where urine is stored until it is excreted. Any changes to your dog's urination habits, or to the urine itself, can alert you to a problem. Prompt veterinary attention is always warranted as bladder infections can spread upwards to the kidneys if left untreated. Due to the varying causes of painful urination, diagnosis is obviously vital so that effective treatment can be started. (Incontinence and other urinary problems of elderly dogs are covered in Chapter 8.)

Common symptoms

Painful and frequent urination is the most common sign. This usually indicates that your dog has cystitis, which means inflammation of the bladder. Cystitis is more common in bitches. You may also notice a change in the colour or smell of your dog's urine; it may be strong-smelling and contain blood.

How to take a urine sample

A fresh urine sample will be very helpful for your vet when assessing a urinary problem. It needs to be fresh, so when you arrive at the surgery ask for a dish and take your dog for a short walk to collect a sample. When your dog urinates, quickly place the dish in the way of the stream. Your vet will only need a very small sample for analysis, so don't worry if you only catch a few drops.

General care for the urinary system

If your dog has cystitis you will always need to encourage him to drink more, as this helps to clear and flush his system. You can do this by adding water to his food and making it a bit mushy for a few days, or soaking his dry food. Also ensure that you give him plenty of opportunities to urinate, by taking him out to the garden frequently.

> **COMMON CAUSES OF URINARY-SYSTEM COMPLAINTS**
>
> - Bacterial cystitis
> - Bladder stones
> - Urinary retention

Complementary treatments for urinary-system complaints

Herbal remedies

Cranberry juice is often used, but make sure it is sugar-free. In addition, Oregon grape, garlic, raspberry leaf and echinacea are all antimicrobial herbs that can help to fight bladder infections. Liquorice and dandelion are indicated for chronic bladder infections.

Homeopathic remedies

Cantharis if there is extreme straining or blood in the urine. Apis Mellifera for dogs that are warm and thirstless. Arsenicum Album for dogs showing straining and restlessness. Sarsaparilla is indicated if the straining is worse at the end of urination, given at 30c potencies twice daily for up to seven days.

THE REPRODUCTIVE SYSTEM

Females

Bitches usually come into season twice a year. If your bitch is not spayed, you need to be aware of a potentially life-threatening condition called 'pyometra', which means infection of the womb. Symptoms can be quite non-specific, but in some cases will include a discharge from the vulva and an increased thirst. So the best advice for any entire bitch that is off-colour is to have her checked over by the vet straight away.

This book does not cover problems concerning pregnancy or parturition.

False pregnancy

False (or pseudo) pregnancy occurs when the bitch seems to be pregnant but isn't. It occurs about two to three months after her last season. Her mammary glands will swell and she may even produce milk. Her behaviour may alter, she may mother toys and socks and seem extra clingy to you. It will usually resolve on its own in two to three weeks. If she has false pregnancies repeatedly and you are not going to breed from your bitch, neutering is usually recommended. It is important to have your bitch checked by the vet and the condition diagnosed if you suspect she is having a false pregnancy.

Complementary treatments for false pregnancy

Homeopathic remedies

Pulsatilla is indicated in bitches that produce a lot of milk, are thirsty, mother a lot of things and want sympathy. Sepia on the other hand is the remedy to use in bitches where there is little milk, and for individuals that seem depressed, but perk up when taken out for a walk. Use 30c and dose twice daily for a week.

Males

See Chapter 8 for information on prostate disease.

THE MUSCULOSKELETAL SYSTEM

The musculoskeletal system comprises the muscles, ligaments, bones and joints. The most common problem affecting your dog's mobility is arthritis. This is inflammation of a joint, causing pain and stiffness. The most common form of arthritis is osteoarthritis, also called degenerative joint disease. This is usually an age-related degeneration of joint cartilage affecting elderly dogs (*see* Chapter 8). Most joint pain occurs due to either loss or damage of cartilage or joint fluid, or to deposition of extra bone within the joint. Any of these situations leads to bone rubbing against bone, as well as a swollen joint capsule, both of which are painful. Joints occur not only in the limbs, but also all along the spine between the vertebrae; arthritis here is called spondylosis. Of course your dog can also suffer from dislocations and fractures, as well as from problems affecting his muscles, ligaments or tendons, all of which can result in pain and lameness.

Your vet will have to check your dog over if he suffers from any sudden onset or ongoing pain and stiffness. He may require x-rays or other diagnostic tests.

Common symptoms

These can range from sudden onset pain and lameness to your dog having long-standing stiffness and reduced range of movement. He may be holding up a leg that is affected, not wanting to bear any weight on it, or he may be lame on it. Arthritis in elderly dogs often presents with initial stiffness on first getting out of bed after a long rest, and with lameness after a long walk.

Routine care for musculoskeletal complaints

In some cases gentle exercise helps as it prevents your dog from seizing up. However, in other cases strict rest will be needed. This is why your dog should be checked over by the vet and a diagnosis made. You will then know what and where the problem is, and how to treat your dog correctly with regard to rest or gentle exercise. Keeping his weight down will be important if your dog does suffer from arthritis, as obesity will put extra strain on his joints.

Complementary treatment for musculoskeletal complaints

Chiropractic treatment
Beneficial in many cases, as it addresses the knock-on effects of altered mobility. For example, where long-term lameness in one limb has caused extra weight or strain on another limb (or along the spine) and hence caused more complex problems than just that of the original injury.

Hydrotherapy and physiotherapy
Often used as part of a rehabilitation programme to help restore function and range of movement.

Acupuncture
A natural form of pain relief that also addresses underlying predisposing factors.

Herbal remedies
Turmeric and Devil's claw are two of the most recognized anti-inflammatory herbs. Comfrey is considered a classic bone and joint repair herb.

Homeopathic remedies
Rhus Tox, Ruta and Arnica: these can be used as a combined remedy (often called 'RRA') for treatment of pain and stiffness that eases up on initial movement. Ruta Grav is the indicated remedy for ligament or tendon strain. For deep muscle injury use Bellis Perennis. Hamamelis is used for bruises, strains and sprains. These can be given at 30c twice daily for several weeks. Don't forget arnica used in a high potency (200c) straight after any injury (to help with shock as well as bruising). After three or four doses change to 30c twice daily.

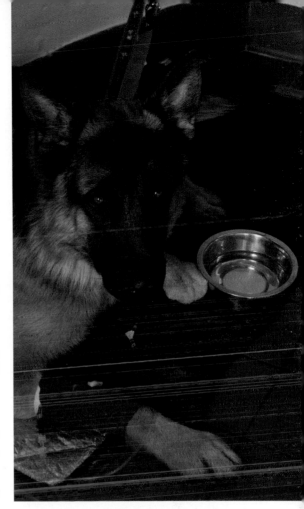
A patient in the veterinary hospital.

Supplements
Antioxidants (vitamins C and E) and glucosamines and chondroitin are indicated for long-term support (*see* Chapter 7).

The spine
Due to the range of possible causes of back problems, and the potential seriousness of some of them, a veterinary check-up is essential. As well as a full physical and neurological examination, your vet may need to perform X-rays or MRI scans in order to make a diagnosis.

The following suggestions for supportive complementary treatments are to be used under veterinary guidance only, and are not intended as sole forms of therapy in serious conditions.

Common symptoms

Back pain can manifest with varied symptoms, ranging from sudden crying when he moves to your dog just seeming off-colour and not himself. There are also the more obvious signs such as stiffness, difficulty getting into or out of the car or up and down steps, lameness or even paralysis. He may also have neurological signs such as stumbling and being unsure of his footing. Your dog may also appear uncharacteristically grumpy or resentful of touch.

Complementary treatments of spinal complaints

Acupuncture

For pain relief and anti-inflammatory action, and for nerve regeneration after injury. Chiropractic treatment may also be indicated.

Homeopathic remedies

Arnica (30c) is indicated for pain and inflammation. RRA, a combination remedy of Rhus Tox, Ruta and Arnica (30c), in

---

COMMON CAUSES OF MUSCULOSKELETAL COMPLAINTS

- Trauma/ injury
- Osteoarthritis
- Developmental problems in young dogs

---

spondylosis, used twice daily for one to two weeks as required. Hypericum (200c), use twice daily for three days for shooting pains associated with nerve-tissue trauma, then reduce to 30c.

THE NERVOUS SYSTEM

The brain and spinal cord make up what is called the central nervous system, while the nerves to the various parts of the body make up the peripheral nervous system. Symptoms of nervous-system disease depend on which part is affected, and range from seizures and tremors, to wobbliness and 'ataxia' (the veterinary term for incoordination).

Routine care for the nervous system

It is wise to remove all potential nervous-system toxins such as air fresheners, household cleaning products, herbicides

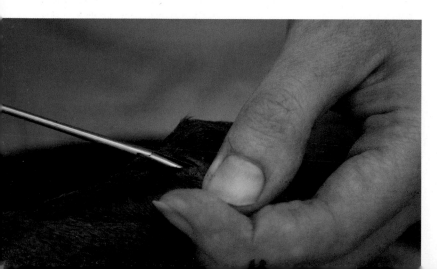

Removing a grass seed from a dog's foot.

**COMMON CAUSES OF
SPINAL COMPLAINTS**

- Trauma or injury
- Intervertebral disc disease
- Spondylosis (degenerative osteo-arthritis of the spine)

---

and garden insecticides from your dog's everyday environment. It is also advisable to stop using any routine insecticide flea-control products, as these are all nervous-system toxins (that is how they kill the fleas).

Seizures

All seizures involve an electrical disturbance in the brain. The most common condition that causes seizures is 'idiopathic epilepsy', which is the diagnosis given when no cause for the seizures can be identified; this can be more common in certain breeds. Seizures can also be due to infections, metabolic diseases, poisoning, cancer, trauma or head injury. Your dog's nervous system is also affected by emotional and mental factors, such as shock and extreme fear.

The following suggestions for supportive complementary treatments are to be used under veterinary guidance only, and are not intended as sole forms of therapy in serious conditions.

Complementary treatments for seizures
Acupuncture
Indicated for treating epilepsy, as it can help to reduce frequency and severity of seizures.

Bach Flower Remedies
Use Rescue Remedy. Also Vervain and Chestnut Bud may be used.

Diet
Add oats to the diet to help calm and settle the nerves. There are some advocates of a low-protein diet for dogs with epilepsy.

Herbal remedies
Skullcap and valerian are well known for their sedating and calming effects. If your dog tends to drink after a seizure then offer him cold chamomile (or valerian) tea.

Homeopathic remedies
Need to be prescribed based on the individual symptoms and can be a highly beneficial form of treatment.

Supplements
B vitamins and L-taurine and L-tyrosine support nerve function. Omega-3 fatty acids are beneficial and support brain function.

First aid for seizures
If your dog has a seizure, do not touch or interfere with him and try to stay calm yourself. Try and protect his head by placing a cushion under it. If necessary you can also drag him by the scruff of the neck away from dangerous places such as the top of the stairs. Never try and dose him with anything or place your hand near your dog's mouth or you risk being

---

COMMON CAUSES OF SEIZURES

- Idiopathic epilepsy
- Infection
- Metabolic disease
- Head injury
- Poisoning

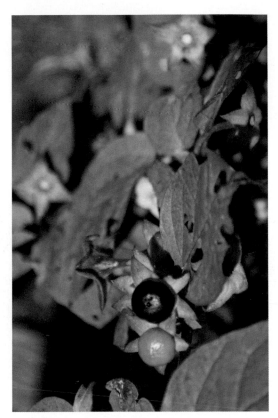

Belladonna (Deadly Nightshade) is a homeopathic remedy for fever.

'Stroke' in old dogs

If you think your dog has had a stroke he is likely to be suffering from something called 'vestibular syndrome'. This is a neurological condition of middle-aged and older dogs, where there is a sudden loss of balance, they may suffer from a head tilt, and sometimes they are unable to stand. Other symptoms include flickering of the eyes, disorientation and wobbliness (ataxia). Of course a veterinary check-up will be important if your dog suddenly shows these symptoms.

Causes of 'stroke' symptoms

There are two types of vestibular syndrome, 'peripheral' and 'central'. The peripheral type is more common and is caused by inflammation in the nerves connecting the middle ear to the brain; the cause of the inflammation is usually not known. Central vestibular disease carries a worse prognosis as it is caused by a problem in the brain itself, for example a tumour. Other causes of these sudden onset neurological symptoms include trauma or injury to the head, and middle or inner ear disease.

General care of vestibular disease

Supportive measures to help your dog recover from peripheral vestibular disease include nursing him at home and hand feeding him, as he often cannot manage to eat from his bowl while his coordination is affected. You can also massage his head and neck to stimulate the circulation and ease any pain; there are many acupressure points in this area.

Complementary treatments for vestibular disease

Acupuncture

To help stimulate the appetite and alleviate nausea and disorientation.

badly bitten (as he can't control his actions during a seizure). If you are indoors, dim the lights and speak to your dog quietly and calmly. You can rub a few drops of Rescue Remedy into the skin at the base of his ears before, during and after a seizure to help relieve anxiety. Always keep a note of the details (times and exact symptoms) of each episode, as this can help you track patterns and potential trigger factors. If it lasts longer than a few minutes get him straight in the car to the vet's, as a seizure that is prolonged can cause permanent brain damage and be life-threatening.

Herbal remedies
Gingko biloba is often indicated as it helps increase blood flow to the brain.

Homeopathic remedies
Causticum (30c) twice daily for one to two weeks.

HIND LIMB WEAKNESS AND INCOORDINATION

Older dogs can suffer from gradual weakness of their hind limbs as they age. However, certain breeds, such as the German shepherd dog, can get a specific neurological condition called 'degenerative myelopathy' (DM), sometimes also known as chronic degenerative radiculomyelopathy (CDRM). This is where the nerve function to their hind legs gradually deteriorates, causing progressive weakness and incoordination as well as incontinence in the later stages. Intervertebral disc disease, spondylosis and certain metabolic diseases can have similar presenting signs. Due to the similarity in symptoms between the various conditions, and yet the very different prognosis and treatment plan for each, a veterinary consultation is essential for any dog showing hind limb weakness or wobbliness.

Complementary treatments
Acupuncture
As well as hydrotherapy and physiotherapy to help maintain function and strength in their back end.

Homeopathic remedies
Conium and Plumbum (can be combined as one remedy), 30c, twice daily for one or two weeks.

Supplements
Omega-3 fatty acids, glucosamines, CoQ10, L-carnitine, acetyl cysteine, vitamins E and B complex.

FIRST AID

The secret is to 'be prepared'. Having a first aid kit for your dog, and knowing how to use what you have in it, is crucial. While minor wounds can be treated at home, if they worsen or your dog is in pain or has any other symptoms, then the vet must see him straight away. There are also courses in canine first aid where you learn cardiopulmonary resuscitation (CPR) etc.

Abscesses
If you want to encourage an abscess to burst, use the homeopathic remedy Hepar Sulph twice daily in 12c. After they have burst bathe abscesses with hypercal solution.

Bites and stings
Apis Mel and Ledum are two homeopathic remedies used for wasp and bee stings to help relieve the stinging and swelling. Give 30c every ten to fifteen minutes until resolved (or for a maximum of five doses).

Burns
Bathe the area under cool running water. Give the homeopathic remedy Cantharis 30c every ten to fifteen minutes until resolved (or for a maximum of five doses). Urtica Urens cream for topical use.

Bruising
Arnica is the number one homeopathic remedy for bruising. Use 200c for two or three doses in acute situations, and then use 30c for twice-daily dosing. Arnica cream can be used on bruises too, but never apply it to open wounds. Topical

yarrow oil applied to a bruise will also help reduce swelling and bruising.

Crushed digits/tail

For injuries involving sensitive nerve endings such as the crush-type injury of your dog's feet getting stepped on or having something dropped on them, or having his tail trapped in a door, use the homeopathic remedy Hypericum (30 or 200c).

Cuts/lacerations

Bathe or flush with hypercal solution and then bandage as necessary. Use hypercal cream topically twice or three times daily.

Shock

Dr Bach's Rescue Remedy, use four drops every ten to fifteen minutes. The homeopathic remedy Aconite (at a high potency, 200c), give two or three doses.

Strains and sprains

Use the homeopathic remedy Ruta Grav (30c) for tendon or ligament injury.

Ripped claws/nails

Clean and bathe them with a solution of hypercal and give the remedy Hypericum by mouth (200c or 30c) as well, to help with nerve pain.

Wounds

Use hypercal solution to bathe wounds. This is a homeopathic antiseptic solution that you can either buy ready made up, or you can make yourself by taking the tinctures of calendula and hypericum and highly diluting them one to twenty with sterile saline. Calendula cream is excellent for helping wounds to heal and should be applied to the area three times a day. Manuka honey can be applied to wounds as a natural antibiotic and antiseptic. Aloe vera is another option; it has a soothing and healing action.

YOUR FIRST AID KIT

- Aconite liquid remedy (200c)
- Aloe vera gel
- Arnica tablets (30c and 200c)
- Bandage (you can also use this as an emergency muzzle)
- Calendula cream
- Hypercal tincture
- Manuka honey
- Rescue Remedy
- Urtica cream
- Witch hazel
- Sterile saline solution
- Blunt-tipped scissors
- Tweezers
- Tick remover
- Thermometer
- Gauze pads
- Roll of adhesive bandage (or get vet wrap from your vet's)
- Collar and lead and dog bowl
- Emergency vet's telephone number taped inside the kit.

USEFUL ADDRESSES

The following are useful sources of further information and suppliers of complementary medicines.

Veterinary homeopathy
The British Association of Homeopathic Veterinary Surgeons (BAHVS), www.bahvs.com

The British Homeopathic Association, Hahnemann House, 29 Park Street West, Luton LU1 3BE Tel. 01582 408 675; www.britishhomeopathy.org

Suppliers of homeopathic remedies
Ainsworth's Homeopathic Pharmacy, 36 New Cavendish Street, London W1G 8UF. Tel. 0207 467 5435; www.ainsworths.com

Freeman's Homeopathic Pharmacy, 18-20 Main Street, Busby, Glasgow G76 8DU, Scotland. Tel. 0845 22 55 1 55; www.freemans.co.uk

Using herbs
The National Institute of Medical Herbalists (NIMH), Elm House, 54 Mary Arches Street, Exeter EX4 3BA. Tel 01392 426 022; www.nimh.org.uk
www.herbalvets.org.uk

Acupuncture
The Association of British Veterinary Acupuncturists, BMAS House, 3 Winnington Court, Northwich, CW8 1AQ. Tel. 01606 786782; www.abva.co.uk

Bach Flower Remedies
The Bach Centre, Mount Vernon, Bakers Lane, Brightwell-cum-Sotwell, Oxon OX10 OPZ. Tel. 01491 834678; www.bach-centre.com

Canine Hydrotherapy
The National Association of Registered Canine Hydrotherapists (NARCH); www.narch.org

Chiropractic
The McTimoney Chiropractic Association, Crowmarsh Gifford, Wallingford, Oxfordshire OX10 8DJ. Tel. 01491 829211; www.mctimoneychiropractic.org

Tellington TTouch Training
Tilley Farm, Timsbury Road, Farmborough, Somerset BA2 0AB. Tel. 01761 471182; www.tilleyfarm.co.uk

To find a rescue dog
The Dogs Trust, 17 Wakley Street, London EC1V 7RQ. Tel. 0207 837 0006; www.dogstrust.org.uk

All about the raw food diet
Raw Food Vets; www.rawfoodvets.com

The professional body for veterinary surgeons
The Royal College of Veterinary Surgeons, Belgravia House, 62–64 Horseferry Road, London SW19 2AF. Tel. 0207 222 2001; www.rcvs.org.uk

FURTHER READING

Fisher, S., *Unlock your dog's potential – how to achieve a calm and happy canine* (David and Charles, 2007)

Fougere, B., *Healthy dogs – a handbook of natural therapies* (Hyland House, 2003)

Hamilton, D., *Homeopathic care for cats and dogs – small doses for small animals* (North Atlantic Books, 1999)

Schwartz, C., *Four paws, five directions – a guide to Chinese medicine for cats and dogs* (Celestial Arts Publishing, 1996)

Tilford, G. and Wulff, M., *Herbs for pets – the natural way to enhance your pet's life* (Bowtie Press, 2009)

ACKNOWLEDGEMENTS

While there isn't enough room to mention everyone who has helped and supported me, I would like to say a special thank you to the following people:

Anne Seawright, Barbara Fougere, Katy Horton, Holly Wallace, Amanda Warner, Tom and Cara Bradley, John Howie, Henrietta Morrison, Jonathan Self, Emma Padfield, Sarah Fisher, Greer Deal, Justin Ainsworth, Tom Goldstein, Tim Sandys and Paula Rogers.

Also a huge thank you to Happy Days Dog Care, The Clifton Vet Practice, The Paw Seasons, The Stoke Bishop Dog Training Club, Vets on White Hart Lane, The UK Wolf Conservation Trust and Canine Partners.

INDEX